DAMNING THE INNOCENT

DAMNING
THE INNOCENT

A History of the Persecution
of the Impotent
in pre-Revolutionary
France

PIERRE DARMON

Translated from the French
by Paul Keegan

VIKING

To my friend, Dr Jean Cohen

VIKING
Viking Penguin Inc.
40 West 23rd Street,
New York, New York 10010, U.S.A.

First American edition
Published in 1986

First published in France as *Le Tribunal de l'Impuissance* by
Editions du Seuil, Paris, 1979. © Editions du Seuil, 1979.

First published in Great Britain
under the title *Trial by Impotence*

LIBRARY OF CONGRESS CATALOGING IN PUBLICATION DATA
Darmon, Pierre, 1939–
Damning the innocent.
Translation of: Le tribunal de l'impuissance.
Bibliography: p.
1. Impotence (Canon law)   2. Marriage—Annulment
(Canon law)   3. Marriage—Annulment—France—History.
I. Title.
LAW   262.9   85-40625
ISBN 0-670-80911-X

Printed in the United States of America by
R. R. Donnelley & Sons Company, Harrisonburg, Virginia
Set in Sabon

Contents

5012892

PUBLISHER'S NOTE

For this translated edition, which is intended for the general
reader, certain cuts have been made, notably technical appendices dealing with juridical matters, and all footnotes and
detailed references. Material of more general interest from
appendices and footnotes has been incorporated into the body
of the text. Readers interested in the full text, including exact
sources for quoted material, are referred to the French edition:
Le Tribunal de l'Impuissance (Editions du Seuil, Paris, 1979).

CONJUGAL DUTY: *by this expression is understood
the marital act as required by law of a spouse
at the request of his or her partner.*

Introduction
Impotence, marriage and the Church

Among the many groups of people who suffered at the hands of the *Ancien Régime* in France – the insane, the poor, sodomites, alchemists and blasphemers – the impotent have long been forgotten.

This book therefore relates the strange and little-known story of all those individuals who, because of a supposedly deficient sexuality, found themselves dragged before the courts and offered up as ransom to the age-old myth of virility. Their story is a pitiful drama of loneliness and silence, a timeless drama which persists in some ways up to the present day. For, whether the trial took place in the full glare of publicity or in the muffled anonymity of a court room, whether the verdict was 'innocent' or 'guilty', the individual accused of impotence was a defenceless victim, crushed in the wheels of indifferent legal and ecclesiastical machinery. His only rights he owed to the benefit of the doubt; because of this, he was provided with a lawyer. But in most cases this afforded no more than a temporary reprieve. It was only a matter of time before he found himself condemned, openly despised and relegated to the ghetto of the morally reprobate.

This book also relates the edifying story of all those who set themselves up as judges of, and zealous crusaders against, impotence, in the name of a notional virility whose functioning was determined by canon law. At some level they were perhaps acting out the same drama of inadequacy as their victims. But who were they, and what hidden forces motivated their behaviour? We can see their early appearance and ascendancy, sanctioned by the Gospel, their activities spurred on by the Church's policy demand for a rising birth rate. And yet the Church Fathers, led by St Paul and St Augustine, were soon to substitute this policy by another, equally peremptory and absolutely imperative: to stamp out sexual lust, the hateful fruit of Original Sin. The evolution of the impotence trial, and its whole justification, proceeded from this command of the Church Fathers.

Behind this holy façade it would be all too easy to detect only the workings of a rather mediocre logic, in which case the celebration of virility and condemnation of impotence could be seen as a form of insurance, a compensatory mechanism. In fact there is a more serious underlying reality. Deep in the shadowy unconscious of every man lurks a terrible fear of castration. The myth of virility can be seen as the sublimation of this anxiety into an abstract form which is the basis of a man's prestige, yet completely beyond his control. The forces that do control it are certainly mysterious. From one day to the next, its happy functions, the tangible proof of male prestige and perfection, can vanish like smoke in the wind, for no apparent reason. It is a cruel state of uncertainty. For all his pride, the virile male is a man trapped by his celebrated and over-estimated body, and the endless escalation of his physical prowess, which, far from reassuring him, plunge him into an infernal spiral of anguish. At any moment, the world which he has built up around himself may disintegrate. For this reason, the trial and condemnation of his impotent fellow men affords him substantial consolation. It serves to idealise his own position, and allows him the opportunity to display his own conformity with the collectively approved sexual norms – a conformity which is statutory, mandatory and of divine ordinance. The priests themselves submit to it, and the Church casts out all those whose virile organ, though sworn to inaction, reveals the slightest anomaly. This paradox is only apparent: for the divine institution, in the image of its Saviour, is compelled to symbolise His perfection which, in this case, is embodied in the most flawless virility.

In these circumstances, the trial assumes the form of a sacrifice in the pagan sense of the term, in which the high-priest or judge unburdens himself of his neuroses by transferring them to his victim. This is the deeper meaning of the impotence trial. It is essentially the product of an ill-assimilated sexuality, and the expression of a confused and murky libido.

From this came the privileged role of the Church in a system devised to channel the impulses of a bruised sexuality and the ragings of unassuaged virility. Throughout the history of these trials, the Church holds the centre of the stage, taking the initiative, activating the chain of guilt. It is true that the lay courts began early on to intervene in the subtle apparatus of repression, and they clearly ended up by playing a dominant role. But what is most significant is that in every trial the Church imposed its presence as the ideological intermediary.

It is true that specific and significant variations in procedure can be traced from one period to another. Up to the middle of the sixteenth century the trials were marked by a certain dignity. 'Fraternal cohabitation' within the framework of a non-consummated marriage was exalted, and the dissolution of marriage considered only as a last resort. But from the end of the century this trend was reversed. Suddenly, the institution of marriage began to deteriorate, and the impotence trial finally came into its own in the atmosphere generated by a sudden explosion of discussion about sexuality. Though in practice sexuality was repressed, it was given a compensatory outlet in verbal outpourings rich in obsessional characteristics. What was in fact remarkable about this phenomenon was not its novelty – for it was already present in the writings of the Church Fathers – but the sudden speeding up of its administrative mechanisms. 'From the end of the sixteenth century,' notes Michel Foucault, 'the "putting into discourse" of sex, far from

undergoing a process of restriction, was on the contrary subjected to a mechanism of increasing excitement.'

Systematic, methodical and incisive, the discourse of sexuality was formulated primarily by the Church. Without the least
scruple, and in the most peremptory manner, the Church
assumed the right to dictate the sexual behaviour of its faithful,
and certain canonists set themselves up as virtuosi in what they
henceforth considered to be a privileged, if not a preferred, area
of expertise. In his researches into the mysteries of the orgasm,
which he scrutinised with rare meticulousness and fanatical
exactitude, Father Sanchez exemplified the new breed of sexual
savants. In his fantastical *De Matrimonio* he accumulated
thousands of questions concerning the finer points of sexual
practice:

Is it lawful to think of another woman while in the act of fulfilling
the conjugal duty?

Is it lawful for each partner to ejaculate independently of the other?
[At this time, female secretions during coitus were thought to be
equivalent to the ejaculation of semen.]

Is it lawful to have relations with a woman without arriving at the
emission of semen?

Is it lawful to help the impotent partner by all manner of fondling
and lures?

Is it lawful to practise intromission elsewhere than in the appropriate orifice?

Nor is this all. Each question leads to another and, by a process
of systematic and labyrinthine extension, the author plunges
into hitherto unsuspected mysteries surrounding the Nativity:
'Did the Virgin Mary emit semen in the course of her relations
with the Holy Spirit?'

The enthusiasm of the canonical discussion of sex was not
lost on some contemporary observers:

These astonishing researches [wrote Voltaire] have been carried out
by no one anywhere in the world, other than our theologians . . . no
peculiarity has escaped their gaze. They have debated every occasion

under which a man might be impotent in one situation and operative in another. They have investigated all that the imagination can devise to further nature's cause; and, with the intention of drawing the line between that which is permitted and that which is not, they have in their earnestness laid bare that which should be cloaked in the secrecy of night.

Like the propaganda of the confessional, or the venomous pastoral letter against nudity of the breasts, the impotence trial constituted one of those privileged arteries leading straight to the heart of the sexual life of the Christian couple. The theological debate which the trials aroused, and the interrogations which they presupposed, bear eloquent testimony to this fact.

Here, the Church did not always stay within the relatively discreet or innocuous bounds of mere language. It took the leap from intellectual onanism to the most exacerbated voyeurism, from theory to practice, with a most indecent agility. The detection of an impotent individual now involved astonishing preliminary tests: from the public demonstrations of 'erection', 'elastic tension' or 'natural motion', and, on occasion, the 'proof of ejaculation', to the incredible 'trial by congress', which involved enacting the marital duties in their entirety in the presence of witnesses. But once again, these procedures were only the superficial structures of a deeper and far more complex machinery of inquisition and repression.

So there is nothing surprising about the violent wave of reaction which swept through the prudish nineteenth century and resulted in the systematic dismantling of an institution which embodied the vices and abuses of the *Ancien Régime*. The disgust with which this gruesome legacy was regarded by the proponents of civil law may easily be imagined. From the beginning of the nineteenth century, therefore, even the mention of impotence was looked upon unfavourably: it no longer existed. In a world preoccupied by good business management, the capitalist bourgeoisie wanted no part of these obtrusive and scandalous trials. A puritanical culture opted for a magnanimous tact in such matters; only the Church still hankered after its pound of flesh.

In actual fact, however, the potential for such accusations still existed, hidden away in obscure manuals on legal medicine. The *Code Civil* itself could not turn a blind eye to the legal consequences of accidental impotence, and this was a dangerous exception out of which new procedures of legal incrimination were formed. From the end of the century these started to encroach upon the activities of the civil courts, sanctioning a return to the days of scandalous fabrications and inquisitions. Clearly impotence as such was no longer the issue. It became customary instead to condemn the 'sexual identity' of the accused, or to cite 'injurious non-consummation' where impotence was regarded as proceeding from a conscious act of will. It was not until very recent times that sexual incapacity, rehabilitated in law, came to entail the annulment of marriage on the grounds of a mistaken choice of partner.

Here, the convergence of civil and ecclesiastical justice is evident. But the paths leading to the same end diverged radically. Today, the civil judge passes sentence according to specific socio-psychological considerations. In a far more systematic manner, the ecclesiastical verdicts always derived from the sacred categorical imperative: the suppression of sexual lust. This explains the relative homogeneity of the impotence trial in the Church courts over a long period of time. For here everything rested upon the inviolable and age-old doctrine of Christian marriage; the impotence trial was primarily an outward expression of this doctrine.

In this sense it can be claimed, without exaggeration, that the Church reduced everything to a question of physical consummation. No doubt the Church would have hotly denied this, by invoking also the union of hearts and souls in the marriage bond. This was in fact an empty myth. Non-consummation acted as a powerful matrimonial dissolvent, whereas marital dissent or incompatibility of temperament were generally regarded as frills.

This idea of marital duty, essentially evangelical in origin, proved haunting and obsessional, and remains to this day the common denominator underpinning all marriages undertaken in a truly Christian perspective. It is around this duty that the entire institution revolves. Without it there is no salvation, and the marriage does not nor has ever existed.

However, it was only around the thirteenth century that the imperative of physical consummation firmly entrenched itself, and subsequently became the official agent of the normalisation of conjugal relations in the classic doctrine of Christian marriage.

In the opinion of the jurist Boucher d'Argis, who, towards the middle of the eighteenth century, established the basic principles of this doctrine, it was essential to contemplate marriage from a triple perspective: natural, political and religious:

In the natural order, marriage is a society constituted by two persons of different sex, whose essence does consist IN THE POWER WITH WHICH THEY DO RECIPROCALLY INVEST THEIR BODIES, to use them in accordance with the ends laid down by the Creator.

This 'society' was therefore a divine institution entrusted with ensuring the propagation of the species, as laid down in Genesis I, 27.

At the same time, the union of man and woman falls within a nobler design which sets it apart from the coupling of animals, for marriage is also the 'union of true minds in conjugal amity'. But Boucher d'Argis is at pains here to emphasise that

this union does not of itself form a marriage, which does also require the union of bodies, in order that the husband may make of her whom he weds bone of his bones and flesh of his flesh, and that husband and wife be henceforth but one flesh (. . .) [Genesis II, 23]

Considered as part of the political order, marriage is a solemn union DESIGNED TO PROVIDE THE STATE WITH LEGITIMATE CITIZENS, and to check the dissoluteness and shame that is the fruit of illegitimate unions (. . .)

Finally, in the religious order, marriage is a sacrament that symbolises for us the intimate and true union of Jesus Christ and his Church (. . .) The outward sign of this sacrament is THE CAPACITY OF THE CONTRACTING PARTIES TO BECOME OF ONE FLESH, the which renders them fit to receive the Sacrament. [Eph. XXV, 5, xxii]

So from every point of view, marriage was determined first and foremost by the physical union of the sexes, and this was the sole focus and point of convergence for theological concern. The Church appears to have been quite unable to rise to a more elevated conception of marital relations. In practice, of course, the Church's conception of marriage was primarily used to curb any unwarranted sexual impulses.

Boucher d'Argis pointed out that marriage was at once

a source of grace and a beneficial sanctuary, where those not fortunate enough to have received the gift of continence should take refuge and find solace for their infirmity.

In the last analysis, this final point is the whole *raison d'être* of Christian marriage. All the writers of the period regarded marriage as a panacea capable of assuaging the torments of the flesh which have tyrannised mankind since the Fall. 'It is better,' wrote the jurist Desmaisons, 'to follow the easy rules that accompany the practice of this legitimate form of incontinence, than to allow oneself to be tormented by those impure flames of desire that consume the celibate's heart.' This viewpoint had already received the unanimous support of the Church Fathers, who likened sexuality to a disease, and considered marriage the lesser of two evils. This produced the indissoluble nature of the bond forged by a consummated union, and the vow of sexual fidelity which united the couple. Any transgression of this destroyed, *ipso facto*, the benefit of the sacrament and cast the sinner into the inferno of illicit sensuality.

However, the dogma of conjugal indissolubility did not come into force immediately. Until the middle of the eleventh century, a general relaxation of morals, together with the absence of specific legislation and penalties, constituted a significant force of inertia. Reluctantly, the Church even came to tolerate – under episcopal supervision – the dissolution of a certain number of marriages which were effectively invalidated either by the extended absence of one of the partners, a sentence of penal servitude, or adultery. It was only towards the beginning of the twelfth century that the dogma of indissolubility finally triumphed, with the reassertion of the classic doctrine contained in the decree of Gratian and the *Sentences* of Peter Lombard. But this framework was so rigid that litigious or difficult cases acquired a startling publicity. To resolve this problem, the Church formally rejected the principle of divorce.

Yet, clearly, there existed a long-standing tradition which was favourable to divorce. As late as the sixteenth century, the jurist Jean Bodin could write – though in a spirit of pure misogyny – that 'there is nothing more pernicious than to constrain unwilling partners to live together', and that it was therefore essential to reinstate the option of repudiating the marriage vows, in the husband's favour, 'so as to curb haughty wives'.

This movement grew considerably in scale during the eighteenth century, when almost all the enlightened spirits of the age denounced the dogma of indissolubility. In 1768 there even appeared a strange pamphlet entitled 'A Dissertation concerning Population'. Behind this demographic façade the anonymous author proclaimed the urgent need to reinstate divorce. Drawing his inspiration from an apocalyptic brand of Malthusianism, he predicted that otherwise France would be entirely depopulated by the year 1838, and argued that the marriages of the old and the sterile, or the forced cohabitation of those couples who were divided by an aversion on the part of one member or by a mutual loathing, had the effect of irreversibly arresting the demographic growth rate: 'All means are valid that serve good ends; reinstate divorce and France will be repopulated.'

By a decree of 28 February 1769, the High Court of Paris ordered that this Dissertation 'be ripped up and burned in public, as striving to establish a system contrary to Reason, Religion and the indissolubility of Marriage, and as containing in addition other matters equally injurious to good Morals.' In his brief, the Assistant Public Prosecutor, Séguier, had announced his intention not to honour with a refutation the product of so weak a mind.

The arguments of the lawyer Linguet in favour of divorce are far more moving, and more substantial, than those of this anonymous author. In a pamphlet published in 1789, Linguet elaborated tirelessly on the theme of the wife sacrificed for social convenience, while very young, to an old, ugly, belligerent, jealous, vindictive, brutal, selfish, unhealthy, miserly husband.

In such cases, a physical separation made it possible to put an end to the conjugal hell without necessarily violating the sacrament itself. In law, this separation 'of bed and table' (*quoad thorum et mensam*, to use the terminology of canon law) differed appreciably from the *separatio sacramentalis*, or divorce proper. The former was generally the result of an offence committed by one of the partners: adultery, heresy (considered by the Church as spiritual fornication), or serious maltreatment. Separation by mutual consent did not exist, and Linguet denounced the hypocrisy of such a system. The judges, he wrote, lack the courage to tell the hapless couple: Go, both of you, and find in other, more suitably adapted marriage ties, the happiness which these have denied you. Instead, the judges counsel them in secret: Avoid each other, do not see each other, and we shall turn a blind eye to the antipathy which divides you.

Moreover, separation worked exclusively in favour of the husband. Alone, he suited himself and regained his freedom, whereas the wife became a temporary or even permanent recluse in a nunnery. Good manners demanded this, according to Linguet:

To regain but the shadow of her former liberty, it is required that she [the woman] plunge herself into an even stricter captivity. The law begins by confining her to a convent, for as long as is necessary to weigh in the balance those reasons which might urge it to release her from under the yoke of her husband.

It was therefore not advisable to commit oneself lightly to such a course. Even then, there remained the problem of finding a 'diriment impediment', an impediment which was considered to nullify the marriage from the beginning, and which was alone able to undo the otherwise indissoluble tie. And not everyone was entitled to such a luxury.

I

The canons of impotence

During the twelfth century, the triumph of the doctrine of indissolubility led to the categorisation of all the diriment impediments to marriage. The number of these varied from one ritual document to another, and such things as insanity, imbecility, and differences of status and fortune were not always considered to be impediments. The Paris ritual listed twelve diriment impediments, while those of Boulogne, Toul, Soissons and Carcassonne listed fifteen. Nor did all impediments have equal importance. For example, if one partner was a serf, this could in theory provide grounds for the annulment of a marriage, but this became increasingly unlikely. Murder, differences in religion, and failure to accord with social norms are only found occasionally in the lists. By contrast, the court records show that far greater importance was accorded to mistaken choice of partner, consanguinity, abduction, secret marriages and marriages between those in holy orders. Cases of bigamy were also extraordinarily frequent.

In addition to diriment impediments, it is worth noting that there were also 'prohibitive impediments' – relatively minor faults such as celebrating a marriage on a feast-day, failure to publish the banns, or murdering a priest. These less serious transgressions did not annul the marriage, whose validity could be confirmed through a new ceremony or the observation of a purificatory penance.

But amongst the diriment impediments proper, archival sources and collections of court records from the sixteenth century onwards reserve pride of place for sexual impotence. And with good reason, for the marriage of a eunuch was seen as an intolerable threat to the doctrine of Christian marriage. It is not surprising, therefore, that theologians should have duly informed themselves about the problems connected with impotence by plunging into the annals of medicine.

Finding a precise definition of impotence was less a matter of medical nicety than an absolute legal and theological necessity. A task of such delicacy could not be undertaken without due consideration. For to declare a marriage invalid – for whatever reason – was to risk sundering a union which the Church had elevated to the ranks of a sacrament. Consequently the definition of impotence rested on a complex forensic apparatus which was the source of all legal proceedings and the constant point of reference for every speech for the defence. At the same time, there was a reluctance to give an exact formulation to an abnormality which placed the accused irrevocably beyond the norms established by God and society. Besides, phallocentric indoctrination was so pervasive that it generated an irresistible need to reaffirm the figure of the virile male, and so the normal and the abnormal were systematically polarised.

At the heart of this dialectic lay a dual objective: to reassure and to incriminate. It was necessary to define the norms within which every man could affirm his potency, and, conversely, to contain from the outset the impotent man within a 'structure of exclusion'. Thus the situation is clarified by being polarised: the impotent will be by definition he who is not potent. The definition offered by Boucher d'Argis exemplifies this process: 'Concerning marriage, we define potency as the aptitude of the contracting parties to fulfil the conjugal duty. Impotency therefore refers to that state which is contrary to this aptitude.' All the specialists resolve the problem by the same negative process, first setting out the eternal trinity which confirms a man's virility: 'erecting, entering, emitting', in the words of the surgeon Guillemeau.

These three canons of virility were expatiated upon at

length, in Latin and in French. To judge a man potent, affirmed the jurist Vincent Tagereau, three conditions had to be fulfilled: 'the first, *ut arrigat*, is erection; the second, *ut vas saemineum referet*, is intromission; the third and last, *ut in vase seminet*, is emission.' Zacchia, the founder of forensic medicine, laid down the same principles, while stressing their close interrelation. The absence of any one of the three faculties constituted a manifest case of impotence. Almost all the jurists were unanimous that erection alone did not suffice, and the lawyer Bouhier unhesitatingly accused the theologian Le Semelier of irresponsibility for asserting the contrary. The eminent Italian expert in canon law, Dominique de Soto, resolved the matter definitively. Pushing the most rigid moral standards to their absolute limit, it was he who classified as impotent those husbands who scattered their semen around the edges of the 'appropriate orifice'. This notion persisted right up to the middle of the twentieth century.

Throughout the eighteenth century the legal definitions of potency and virility underwent hardly any changes. 'For a man to be considered potent,' wrote Garat, with a little more imagination than other commentators,

it is needful that the physical person of the woman upon whom his heart has set its choice should inspire in his blood that heat and motion which, by arousing such desires, endows the organs of man with a motion and extension which they do in no sense possess while in their tranquil state . . . It is further required that he contain within him the generative seed and that he be capable of sowing the same within his wife at the moment of their sexual conjunction.

However, the complexities of impotence were ill-adapted to so rigid a schematisation. Jurists realised this, but given their reluctance to call into question the three fundamental definitions of virility, they inevitably resorted to an increase in the variables according to which impotence was measured. 'It is exceedingly difficult,' expounded the lawyer Héricourt, 'to determine whether impotency be absolute or respective, whether it be perpetual or whether it disappears after a certain term, whether it exists prior to marriage or arises of a sudden through some complication following the wedding.'

This conveys the predicament in which the jurists found themselves. Because of its variety, the phenomenon of impotence did not lend itself to hasty generalisations or Manichean choices. The task of the judge was a delicate one. Before reaching a decision, he would have to establish with the utmost care the exact legal status of each case, for impotence did not always constitute grounds for annulment. The theologians were the first to integrate the various forms of impotence within a precise legal structure, under the heading 'De Frigidis et Maleficiatis'.

Natural, perpetual and incurable impotence constituted the diriment impediment *par excellence*. It automatically entailed the annulment of a wrongfully contracted marriage, and the husband was forbidden to remarry.

Accidental impotence, resulting from some mutilation or illness, did not necessarily constitute grounds for annulment – whether it was curable or not.

Relative impotence only occurred as a reaction to a certain type of partner. An example might be a man whose appetites were normal when their object was a widow, but who was incapable of experiencing the least sexual arousal in the presence of a virgin. In that case his marriage would be annulled, but the verdict would carry a discretionary permission to remarry – for his second wife he would only be allowed to choose a widow.

Respective impotence signified a mutual physical incapacity in a couple: the partners might be individually potent, but respectively impotent. Their marriage would be dissolved and they would each receive permission to provide for themselves elsewhere, as their natural proclivities dictated. In this case the skill of the judge consisted wholly in his ability to detect any collusion between the partners and in recognising a disguised divorce when he was presented with one.

'Frigidity by evil spell' was thought to be caused by drinking some sort of potion, by the casting of an evil spell or charm, or by the 'ligature or *nouement d'aiguillette*'. (The *aiguillette* was a thin ribbon or string attaching the breeches to the doublet. *Nouer l'aiguillette* means, literally, to knot or tangle this ribbon, but the idiomatic meaning of *nouement d'aiguillette* was to cause impotence by casting an evil spell.)

Female impotence was in the majority of cases connected with an obstruction or excessive narrowness of the vagina (impotence *ex clausura uteri aut nimia arctitudine*, as the texts called it). This might be deemed a diriment impediment, depending upon whether it was congenital or accidental, perpetual or temporary, incurable or curable.

There was a temporal aspect to marital impotence: if it was proved to exist prior to the marriage, the outcome was invariably an annulment; if it appeared afterwards, there were no grounds for annulment.

Yet all these classifications were not able to afford a permanent solution to the problem. Each category of impotence had its own ramifications, its own exceptions and ambiguous cases.

'Frigidity' was the most frequent but the least clearly defined type of impotence, for the simple reason that it resisted all attempts at a rational explanation. Men who were healthily formed and endowed with normal sexual attributes, but who were unable to achieve erection, were referred to as frigid. Boucher d'Argis stated the case quite plainly: 'That blemish which we term frigidity is a falling off of vigour and a kind of feebleness of disposition that proceeds neither from dotage nor from any passing ailment.' A delicate and uncertain matter to diagnose, frigidity was the source of a hypothetical and open-ended forensic debate. During the seventeenth and eighteenth centuries, the cases of De Langey, De Gesvres, Le Gros and François Michel were widely discussed and gave rise to passionate conflicts of opinion. These husbands were perfectly formed sexually and yet their wives complained that they never enjoyed the benefits thereof. For the authorities such cases were especially difficult, since they indicated that the possession of normal sexual attributes did not necessarily imply a capacity to achieve erection, intromission and ejaculation. This 'occult impotence' – to use the expression of Vincent Tagereau – caused the progressive deterioration in the forensic procedures connected with marital dissolution. When a simple examination of the genitals proved insufficient, nobody could resist the development towards 'proof of erection' and, finally, trial by sexual congress.

In the case of eunuchs – those afflicted by 'overt impotence' (Tagereau) resulting from some congenital malformation – there were fewer problems. In its fullest sense, the term 'eunuch' means a complete absence of genitals. Occasionally these do exist, but with some flagrant anomaly. Tagereau reported the case of a man 'possessed of two penises, each hindering the other', of another whose testicles were situated above his penis, and of a third 'who had a penis the size of a wart and testicles that of two peas, hardly discernible.'

The contempt in which these unfortunate individuals were held by the general public reduced them to the level of outcasts or monsters. 'They bear the mark of their ignominy upon themselves,' wrote the theologian Fevret. 'How might we consider them to be whole, since this blemish in them is so considerable, and what reasons might induce us to believe them fit for marriage?' The verdict of Sébastien Roulliard was even more savage: 'These castrates are incapable of progeny, and we do take it as given that it is these which either sex is accustomed to hold in abomination, and whom the Greeks termed half-men or half-women, neither men nor women.' In their hatred of eunuchs, some went so far as to call them creatures of the devil. According to the lawyer Peleus, 'spados [eunuchs] are incubate demons, for which reason, in the manner of those spirits that have relations with women, their substance is colder than the icy wastes of Scythia, and does spoil the reproductive faculty that women possess by nature.'

As a result, eunuchs found themselves outcasts, rigidly ostracised by ecclesiastical and civil legislation. Around the figure of the eunuch there extended a web of prohibitions which excluded him completely from society. It is an inexplicable paradox, to say the least, that the Church should reject all those whose sexual anatomy manifested the slightest anomaly [Dt XXIII], and that the articles of canon law should prescribe a scrupulous and intimate physical examination of candidates for the monastic orders. The fact is that phallocentrism and sexual taboo were perfectly compatible in the context of the Church. Not that civil institutions lagged behind in this respect – eunuchs were prohibited from admittance to public office, and it seems that for a considerable part of the sixteenth century even men who possessed only one testicle were subject to discrimination.

In certain cases, however, eunuchs did pose problems which the authorities found it difficult to resolve. Although deprived of testicles and unable to ejaculate, they were often able to achieve an erection of satisfactory dimensions. In addition, they could possess 'all those other attributes of true men, a voice that is no wise effeminate, a spirit that is no wise dulled, and a growth of hair that differs not from other men.' The question was whether such individuals, whose physical appearance was if anything rather attractive, should be classified as eunuchs.

Until the early seventeenth century, doctors of the Church and jurists sheltered behind the authority of Panorme and, despite some dissent, usually ruled in favour of these ambiguous individuals. However, while the latter were allowed to marry, they could by the same token be declared impotent (because of their inability to emit semen) as soon as their wives – in whose discretion the matter rested – saw fit to appeal for an annulment.

However, two events which occurred in rapid succession – the decree of Pope Sixtus V (1587) and the lawsuit involving D'Argenton (1601) – were to cast new doubts upon the fate of these problematic eunuchs.

On 27 June 1587, Sixtus V drafted a brief for the benefit of his legate in Spain. 'At the present time,' he wrote, 'the women of this country do willingly marry men that, usurping the title of "husband", hold up to ridicule the sacrament of marriage and abandon themselves to a fallacious counterfeit of its holy mysteries. In reality, such unions constitute abominable refinements of debauchery and bear in them the brand of sin and the seeds of damnation.' For these reasons, Sixtus V ordered the mandatory dissolution of these guilty marriages, whether the partners concerned wished it or not. This edict seems to have applied to the whole of Europe, and Spain was probably the last bastion of liberalism. 'Sixtus V did write to his ambassador in Spain, where they do still tolerate the marriages of eunuchs . . .' wrote Gerbais in his *Treatise on the Power of the Church* in 1646. Prior to this, annulment had always been a matter of 'private right', but the brief of 1587 accorded impotence the status of a 'public impediment', which was justified on the grounds of avoiding the depravity caused by unions of this kind.

Ultimately, the decree of Sixtus V marked a definite worsening of the fate reserved for the 'impotent', by putting an end to the passive liberalism of some authorities and courts. From now on, repression was to become more pronounced, and it achieved its height in the D'Argenton affair. But here the sword was to prove double-edged.

In 1595 the Baron d'Argenton married Magdeleine de la Chastre, 'a young maiden of noble and ancient lineage'. According to Sébastien Roulliard, the marriage was consummated on the wedding night and the bloodstained sheet handed over to an inquisitive entourage. For four years of married life the couple 'rendered each to the other their conjugal debt'. However, 'the faculties of the wife were of an unreasonableness such as to render her easily susceptible to gloomy phantasies.' Besides her susceptibility to the deceptive promptings of a 'frivolous imagination', Magdeleine de la Chastre was also subject to the harmful influence of her mother, and she became convinced that her husband was impotent. She lodged a suit and the case came before the ecclesiastical judge of Sens, who promptly ordered an inspection to be made of the Baron's genitals. The report specified that D'Argenton 'had no visible cullions [testicles], but as if a purse without sovereigns, the which did withdraw inside his person when he turned over, in such fashion that he had nothing left him but his member, and even this being far smaller than is customary among men.'

The Baron protested. His testicles existed but were 'hid within'. He requested trial by congress. The ecclesiastical court refused: the absence of visible testicles was considered to be of itself sufficient proof, and the modesty of Magdeleine de la Chastre could therefore be spared a trial. In reply the accused turned to the Primate of Lyon. The verdict was confirmed, as it was when he then addressed himself to Rome. Refusing to admit defeat, he launched a new appeal to the Holy Father, asking him to place the affair in the proper hands. This time the suit was granted, only for Magdeleine now to lodge an 'appeal as against an injustice'.

By this time, the hypothetical testicles had become famous, and were the subject of a very lively philosophical and forensic controversy.

The Baron's lawyer, Du Marché, cited the testimony of

surgeons and theologians who affirmed – with relevant evidence at the ready – that 'apparent testicles' were by no means necessary implements for 'tilling the soil of love'. In his own defence D'Argenton exclaimed: 'I am in no wise a castrate, for I have a bearded chin and my voice is not shrill but resembles that of other men, being strong and manly.' And he added that it was common knowledge 'that beards derive from the abundance of that humour which does flow from the front of the head and is drawn downwards by the force of the cullions [testicles], which do attract the prolific matter of generation . . .' This is evidently why, when 'the agreeable and itchy promptings of love do hasten coitus, then the beard does likewise and at the same time grow.'

The rhetoric was in vain, for in 1600 D'Argenton lost the case. Nevertheless, the affair as such was merely beginning. D'Argenton instructed a lawyer from Melun, Sébastien Roulliard, to prove that despite appearances his elusive testicles definitely existed.

Sébastien Roulliard took up and extended the arguments of Du Marché. Rising to the level of philosophical principles, and employing all sorts of sophistries, he demonstrated that concealment always plays an important part in human affairs. Thus Louis XI was able to suppress the revolt of one of his most distinguished nobles all the more effectively since he had wind of the affair through a witness who – on the analogy of D'Argenton's testicles – was concealed behind an arras when the plot was being hatched. To deny the existence of testicles because they happened to be concealed was to deny by the same token the liver, the lungs, the heart, and so on. Several species – fish, for example – have their testicles concealed inside their bodies. According to Roulliard, this made them 'only the more apt and hot for coitus' (a notion deriving from Aristotle).

Moreover, the possession of testicles was not a necessary prerequisite of erection. Roulliard argued that, on the contrary, they controlled the excesses of sexual lust, serving as 'gates full of sinuous twists and turns to hinder the rapid course of the semen, holding it in check and in a state of suspension . . . and giving an even keel and balance to the boat which does ply back and forth above . . . mounting an armed guard at the entry of the spermatic vessels, so as to prevent them from precipitating themselves all at once in a single mob' (after Paré and Aristotle).

The actual verdict nevertheless remained unaffected by these arguments, and, on 3 February 1604, the Baron d'Argenton died without ever having cleared his name. But his death made it possible to resolve once and for all a ticklish problem of forensic medicine. The whole of Paris rushed to be present at the autopsy of his body, which took place 'in the presence of doctors, surgeons and divers gentlefolk'. To everyone's amazement, 'his two cullions, that nature had concealed from view, showed themselves, and, upon being anatomised, were found to be in all respects similar to those of other men.' D'Argenton was posthumously declared potent, and the Faculty of Medicine of Paris pronounced by decree 'that for the purposes of engendering offspring, it is not requisite that testicles be present in the scrotum of a man, provided nevertheless that he display other and sufficient marks of virility.'

This ruling established a precedent. But it seems not to have been followed consistently, at least to start with. Thus, on 5 January 1607 the High Court of Paris submitted, on appeal, a verdict in favour of Claudine Godefroy 'that there was just cause that she do not forego the celebration of her nuptials, since the doctors and surgeons affirmed in their report that the man had but one testicle, though they added that he was notwithstanding capable of engendering.'

Three types of impotence came to be recognised: accidental, respective and relative impotence.

Accidental impotence was defined as afflicting men who were by nature well-formed. It resulted from an injury, an illness or a surgical operation. It constituted a diriment impediment only when the accident had occurred prior to marriage, but had no power to dissolve a marriage if the accident occurred after the nuptials.

Not all accidents of this kind necessarily led to impotence. At the beginning of the seventeenth century, the surgeon Guillemeau noted that the removal of one or even of both testicles did not put a definitive end to sexual relations.

For this reason, a decision of the ecclesiastical court of Paris nonsuited a woman who had requested the dissolution of her marriage, and 'condemned her to return to her husband.' The latter was 'possessed of but a single testicle, the left one having been removed . . . the which fact we [the experts] deem not to constitute an obstacle such as to impede the power of generation.' In another case of accidental impotence, the bone of contention was a venereal disease contracted by one Nicolas Herbin prior to his marriage. His wife, Marie Plansson, had been granted an annulment by the ecclesiastical judge of Paris. But the husband, arguing that the disease was only temporary, brought the case before the High Court, which quashed the verdict of the ecclesiastical court.

The leniency of judges in matters of accidental impotence is by no means surprising, for no stigma is attached to the individual who has such a misfortune. The abnormality was regarded as strictly circumstantial, and had none of the overtones of a monstrosity which disturbed and defied the laws of nature, society and religion. The categories of respective and relative impotence were regarded in the same light. However the latter, left to the largely subjective appraisal of judges and doctors, raised problems of a more delicate nature.

Unlike absolute or perpetual impotence, which was unaffected by the choice of marital partner, respective and relative impotence were intermittent and selective. Moreover, writers on the subject tended very often to confuse these two last categories. Bouhier was not the first to diagnose a case of 'respective' impotence as one of 'relative' impotence. Boucher d'Argis was far more exact in his definitions. 'Respective impotence,' he wrote, 'can be understood as proceeding from a mutual abnormality in the couple.' Thus the protuberant stomachs of a husband and wife may hinder any form of sexual relations, but this disability will vanish as soon as each finds a partner more adapted to his or her physical contours. In such cases annulment was the obvious course to take.

Relative impotence, on the other hand, affected only one of the partners, the size of whose sexual organs was disproportionate in relation to the commonly agreed norms. As early as the thirteenth century, the theologian Hostiensis had raised this problem in the context of canon law. According to him, Avicenna had already remarked that certain women, tiring of the undersized attributes of their husbands, would go elsewhere in search of more substantial pleasures. Variations on this theme included penises too large or too weak to force the cramped antrum of a virgin, and certain women being too narrow to allow the penetration of a well-proportioned member. In all of these circumstances the dissolution of the marriage was considered necessary.

But, given the vagueness of the legal definitions of relative impotence, it was inevitable that abuses and misinterpretations were to become a common feature of the canonical assizes. In this way it became accepted that certain men who were impotent when confronted with virgins could become virile when partnered with widows. From this arose the custom of dissolving marriages and appending bizarre injunctions forbidding the husband to remarry a virgin but permitting him to marry a widow. In 1610, Vincent Tagereau denounced this practice as contrary to the spirit of Canon law: 'This distinction between aptitude with a widow and ineptitude with a maid, which does pass today as the semblance and pretext for the majority of separations, is not to be found in any canon or decree.' The dictionary of canon law compiled in 1761 by Durand de Maillane further illustrates the legal uncertainty which surrounded the concept of relative impotence. 'Saint Thomas does not believe that there be such a thing as respective impotence [the term has been wrongly used in place of relative impotence]; Saint Anthony strongly claims the contrary; and Father Alexander remarks that in France they do follow the sentiment of Saint Anthony.'

The collections of court records frequently allude to this category of impotence. On 24 December 1613, Magdeleine de Charbonnier was granted a separation from Jean Faure 'on the ground that her said husband's virile organ was so large as to be beyond any virgin to sustain it.'

One man whose marriage had been dissolved on the grounds of impotence remarried a widow. But unfortunately he proved to be as lacking in inspiration with the widow as with the virgin, and the second marriage was in turn annulled. The unsatisfied widow claimed damages. However, on 8 February 1610 the High Court of Paris nonsuited her and ordered her to pay costs, thereby underlining the entirely equivocal character of these authorisations for selective marriage.

Moreover, the notion of relative impotence was responsible for situations which made complete nonsense of the institution of marriage. Thus one couple 'of illustrious lineage' had for some time been living in conjugal harmony. The wife was 'of a most eminent virtue' – her husband had never touched her. Of a philosophical disposition, however, he had succeeded admirably in adapting to the situation in which, for whatever reason, they found themselves. Nor was this surprising, for he 'maintained in his house divers concubines by which he had fathered several children.' After twelve years of this regime, his wife finally came to realise that her household was in certain respects infringing the laws of Christian marriage. She retired to her mother's, from whom she learnt that she was in fact a virgin and that 'her husband was impotent with regard to herself though not with regard to other women.' The marriage was subsequently dissolved 'with permission granted to either party that each was entitled to marry another.'

This nefarious relationship is less surprising than the casual manner in which Bouhier describes it. That this austere magistrate should have seen no more in this story than a footnote to his argument speaks volumes about the fragility of marriage in the institutions of the *Ancien Régime*.

Accidental impotence could afflict a man as the result of an injury, an illness or an operation. Jurists referred to the causes of such impotence as 'violent'. But another type of impotence was recognised: impotence thought to have supernatural, magical or evil causes.

'Frigidity through evil spell' was one of the most fertile sources of theological and legal speculation. Paradoxically, the collections of court records make almost no mention of this formula. When, in the sixteenth century, Jean Papon referred to a verdict which cited impotence through supernatural causes, he proved only to be an exception to the rule. There were occasional cases of those accused of impotence defending themselves by blaming their condition upon magic spells. But the judges, on the look-out for opportunism, nearly always remained sceptical. If pressed, the defendant would accuse his wife of being behind the spell. In 1603, Jacques de Sales, a gentleman of Boissans, claimed before the ecclesiastical judge of Rodez that an evil spell instigated by his wife had stripped him of his virility. The marriage was dissolved, but the partners received permission to remarry. Neither Puymisson, who mentioned this case in his *Plaidoyez*, nor any of the jurists who subsequently cited it, made any attempt to establish whether the dogma of indissolubility had in fact been flouted and the evil spell used as a mere pretext.

The above was, admittedly, an extremely rare case. In 1725, Pierre Decombes, clerk to the Ecclesiastical Court of Paris since 1701, claimed that he had never encountered a reference to 'frigidity through evil spell' in any of the impotence trials at which he had assisted. Moreover, he added that there was no trace of this formula in the minutes of the clerk's office. Forty years later, the lawyer Bouhier mourned the decline of the notion of impotence by evil spell. 'In this matter,' he wrote, 'the credulity of some and the incredulity of others have been pushed too far.'

The ill repute in which 'frigidity through evil spell' was held from the sixteenth century onwards is somewhat paradoxical, given that it was an age of witchcraft epidemics. The classic works on demonology – Sprenger, Delrio, Bodin, De Lancre – are the authoritative sources, and they savagely demonstrate the gravity with which such visitations were normally regarded. The magistrates, themselves victims of this psychotic atmosphere, listened avidly to the most far-fetched reports, denunciations and confessions, and they branded those who displayed the least scepticism in such matters as the devil's henchmen. So, within the context of the Church courts, the bizarre magic spells which supposedly overcame the impotent husband did not arouse any particular emotional response.

Some accounts of the *nouement d'aiguillette* or 'tying the breeches-ribbon', as these spells were known, are bizarre indeed. In *Demonology of Witchcraft* in 1580, Jean Bodin writes:

Of all the foulnesses of the black arts, there is none more common in every part of the land, nor hardly more pernicious, than the impediment that is given to those who marry, that is called 'lier l'aiguillette', even up to young children who do make of this a regular trade, with such impunity and licence that they are not even at pains to conceal it, and many do boast of it quite openly.

In his *Treatise on Superstitions* of 1679, the Abbé Thiers describes some of the many forms that the *nouement d'aiguillette* could take. According to him, the makers of such spells are:

> Those who do pronounce three times the name and the surname of the new-wed couple, forming on the first time a loose knot, and on the second time pulling it a little tighter, and the third time knotting it quite tight . . .
> Those who do make a knot in a breeches-ribbon or a string saying 'Ribald' and making for the first time a cross; then saying 'Nobal', the while making a second cross and a second knot; and at last 'Varnabi' while making a third cross and a third knot, during the time that the Priest . . .
> Those who do tie up the virile part of a wolf, the while reciting the name of a new-wed husband and his bride . . .
> Those who do take a hair of a . . . and a hair of a . . . and do tie them together with all their strength, and with many knots, during the time that the Priest do say to the man and maid: *Ego in matrimonium vos conjugo* . . .

In actual fact, even if the most intransigent jurists unreservedly admitted the principle of 'frigidity through evil spell', they proved considerably more circumspect when it came to assessing its effects. Knowing that outwardly nothing distinguished natural from supernatural frigidity, when in doubt they preferred to pronounce on the side of the former. Besides, without necessarily sharing Montaigne's scepticism in matters of witchcraft, they recognised, like him, that the imagination often engenders 'that casual faintness, which so unseasonably surpriseth passionate lovers, and that chillness which by the power of an extreme heat doth seize on them in the very midst of their joy and enjoying.' In the mid-eighteenth century Boucher d'Argis, writing as a demonologist about the sixteenth century, did not underestimate the significance of psychological factors in the domain of sexual relations. In his opinion, the imagination was responsible for these 'supposed evil spells', and the fear of such spells was in itself sufficient to suspend the virile faculties of a perfectly healthy man. 'In an enlightened age such as our own, and above all in the High Court of Paris, we invest but little faith in these *nouements d'aiguillettes*, for we have often known them to be illusory and to derive commonly from natural causes, as in some potion administered, or from the effects of a blighted imagination.'

This view was endorsed by the forensic surgeons. The re-nowned Zacchia, without going so far as to deny the exist-ence of evil spells, was careful to take account of the inhibitions which, under certain circumstances, could affect couples. 'Im-potency,' he noted lucidly, could proceed 'from timidity or modesty, from an overweening love, or equally from a relent-less hatred of the woman whom a husband has been forced to marry against his will.'

Above all, the argument for frigidity by evil spell was far too attractive to couples intent upon finding a loophole in the doctrine of indissolubility, given that annulments based upon this pretext usually entailed a permission for both partners to remarry. This fact alone may have been the reason for its disfavour in the courts.

Under these circumstances, it seems difficult to explain the contradictory attachment of jurists to a concept which had become completely hypothetical. Yet as late as 1756, Boucher d'Argis devoted an important chapter in his major work to the theme, and Le Semelier had done the same in 1713. In fact, the straightforward rejection of a theory upon which depended a large part of the power and prestige of the constituent bodies was naturally somewhat difficult for them. So, long after the Edict of Colbert in 1682 officially marked the end of witchcraft trials in France, learned discussions on the subject of frigidity by evil spell continued, as nostalgic remnants of a golden age.

The casting of spells to cause impotence has a long history. In the ancient world, the pharaoh Amasis was reputedly a victim. Brunhilda put a charm upon her son, Thierry, King of Burgundy, who became incapable of sexually enjoying his wife, Hermemberge. Ludovic Sforza 'unmanned by means of an evil spell' his nephew Gian Galeazzo, in order to acquire control of the Milanese by depriving him of heirs. These are merely a few examples from the roll-call of historical victims of the evil spell.

The first to consider this phenomenon in the context of canon law was Hincmar, archbishop of Rheims, in the ninth century. In one of his epistles, he states that if God considers it right to allow Satan, through the medium of his earthly henchmen, to prevent the consummation of a marriage, the couple should be exhorted to confess their sins and to practise the virtues of humility, almsgiving, penitence and prayer – and that if, in spite of everything, the impotence persists, the marriage should be dissolved. Drawn from these reflections and incorporated into the decree of Gratian in the twelfth century, the Canon *Si per sortarias* (53,I) became a permanent reference point for jurists and theologians. For legal purposes, this canon assimilated impotence caused by evil spells to a form of accidental impotence. But whether it was to be regarded as permanent or temporary remained unclear, and became the subject of a remarkable controversy.

According to some authorities, such as Pope Innocent IV (1243–54), it was essential at all costs to refrain from declaring an annulment on such grounds: an evil spell was never permanent, and could be lifted by whoever had placed it, or neutralised through prayers or the intercession of divine grace. According to others, evil spells were binding until death, unless the instigator of the spell happened to die before the victim. Furthermore the sexual frustration resulting from this perpetual impotence could lead on either side to adultery or even murder. It was on the basis of such reasoning that a decree of

Pope Honorius III (1216–27) ranked impotence caused by evil spells among the diriment impediments. Again, it was essential that the condition exist prior to the marriage. If it manifested itself only after the wedding, there was no reason to assume that the validity of a correctly undertaken wedding rite had been compromised. Thus the humanitarian argument was ridiculed, and the wife, exposed to the temptations of adultery and the murderous rages of an impotent husband, found herself deliberately sacrificed to the formalities of canon law – particularly if the spell was cast a few minutes after the wedding ceremony. To aggravate matters, evil spells were nearly always cast at the time of the marriage or afterwards.

We must also remember the relativity which was an essential characteristic of impotence caused by an evil spell. As a manifestation of evil, it was logical that the spell – though it might prevent lawful sexual intercourse between marital partners – should not affect the virile faculties of the husband when he exercised these sinfully with another woman. Conversely, there did exist the rare 'good spell', by which the marital partners were rendered impotent when they attempted to commit adultery. Hostiensis reported the case of a certain Count who, for more than thirty years, found it impossible to enjoy any woman other than his wife.

Fundamentally, supernatural impotence, like natural impotence, involved the annulment of marriage – at least in theory. But the husband, whose impotence was in such cases only relative, would therefore remain free to remarry. This was the reason for the extreme caution of the judges that has already been mentioned, and their reluctance to grant annulments on the grounds of supernatural impotence. At the same time it would be misleading to assume that the phenomenon masked only devious intentions on the part of the litigants. For belief in this phenomenon was sometimes genuine, and, most importantly, it lay at the heart of an obsessional climate of opinion

which had outlived its official disgrace in the courts by many
years.

The caution of the ecclesiastics and jurists was all the more
justified in that a host of superstitions surrounded the notion of
supernatural impotence. The Church seems to have advised
neutralising evil spells by 'prayers, tears and penance' in vain.
These innocuous though demanding remedies hardly inspired
the faithful, who were more receptive to the idea of applying
spells to cast out spells. In this light, the warnings issued by the
ecclesiastics are more understandable. 'When therefore this
evil befalls us, we must strive to guard against having recourse
to the demon or his ministers, that is, to the instigators of these
evil spells, such a remedy being an even greater evil,' wrote
Gerbais in 1646. But the fear of such spells remained so deeply
rooted that people not only attempted to allay them but also
to prevent them, by resorting to all sorts of superstitious
practices.

From the sixteenth century onwards, canonical legislation
tried without success to check these tendencies. The law was
constantly infringed because it was so frequently updated. If
we are to judge by the rate at which synodal decrees were
passed, this climate of obsession seems to have reached the
peak of its intensity between 1579 and 1585. In 1579, the
Assembly of Melun forbade marriages to be held at night for
fear of evil spells, and in 1581 the Synod of Rouen instructed
parish priests to bless all marriages unreservedly, in order to
thwart attempts at evil spells and to reassure the faithful. In
1583, the Synod of Rheims determined that nocturnal or
clandestine marriages were sinful. In the same year, the Synod
of Tours denounced the custom of throwing the wedding rings
to the ground to ward off spells. In 1585, the Synod of Aix
recommended that parish priests should protect couples by
advising them to make a full confession at least three days
before the consummation of the marriage. Finally, diocesan

statutes and rituals contained a single condemnation against those who cast evil spells and the superstitious practices designed to counteract them.

In effect, the perpetual reminders of danger seem to have nurtured an obsessional fear, which in turn generated lasting inhibitions. Victims would stop at nothing to be released from the evil by which they considered themselves to be possessed. 'Whether it be God or the Devil that delivers them,' wrote the Abbé Thiers, 'is something that concerns them but little, so long as they be delivered.' From these reactions came the success of superstitious practices. Some of these were quite astonishing, and Thiers enumerates them only to denounce their widespread use and sacrilegious nature. For example:

Wait until another couple do marry, and when the priest does place the ring upon the wife's finger, cut the knot and cast it upon the fire or tread it under foot, with the words *Tibi soli* . . . [In this way the victims of a spell could get rid of it by transferring it to another newly wed couple]

Make the newly wedded couple stand all naked on the paving stones or on earth; make the husband kiss the big toe of his wife's left foot; make each give the other the sign of the cross with their heels, and again with their hands . . .

When the newly wedded couple are about to lie together on the first night of their marriage, make them write on a note the words *Omnia ossa mea* . . . and on another, *Quis similis* . . . then bind the first note to the right thigh of the husband, and the second note to the left thigh of the wife . . .

Broach a barrel of white wine, from which none has yet been drawn, and pour the first wine that comes out over the ring that was given to the wife on her wedding day . . .

Piss through the keyhole of the Church in which your marriage rites were held. Some hold that for this method to have all the success that is desired, one must piss into this hole on three or four mornings in succession.

But perhaps the most efficacious of all remedies was that administered by:

a certain officer of the ecclesiastical court of Châteaudun. When a newly wedded couple came to him saying they were prey to evil spells, he did lead them to his garret, tie them facing each other to a post, the post being however between them, and did whip them repeatedly with a birch; after which he untied them and did leave them together for the night, giving each twopenny worth of bread and a chopin [half a pint] of good wine and locking them in together. The following morning he went to open the door upon the stroke of six, and did find them healthy, sprightly, and on most intimate terms.

A second wedding ceremony seems to have enjoyed a certain popularity with couples hoping to neutralise the influence of evil spells. But, according to the Abbé Thiers, the practice was denounced by the synodal statutes of the dioceses as 'crass ignorance, a vulgar error, a manifest abuse, impiousness, sacrilege, the devil's work, and an outrage to the holy sacrament.' However, some ecclesiastics saw the practice as nothing but an innocent remedy against evil. Father Théophile Raynaud even claimed that after a second wedding ceremony a gentleman named Monclus had fathered three children by his wife, with whom he had been unable to achieve orgasm for fifteen years.

To ward off evil spells, some couples would put salt in their pockets or in their shoes, others would marry at night or in secret, have several wedding rings blessed at the same time or only place the ring up to the first joint of the wife's finger.

Ultimately, pre-marital consummation seems to have been the most enjoyable way of protecting oneself against the sudden discovery of impotence through evil spell. This ruse was probably not the fruit of any subtle theological reasoning, and many libertines must have used it to further their own opportunistic ends. In 1664, one Hercule Bouvard wanted to marry his fiancée, Marie Heard, who appeared to be somewhat hesitant. So he claimed before the ecclesiastical judge that marriage was unavoidable because he had been granted 'certain liberties' by the young woman. When it was pointed out to him that because of this act of fornication he was excluded from the holy sacrament of marriage, he calmly replied 'that what he had done was not performed out of lechery but to prevent the casting of an evil spell, which he had in the past experienced, to his great displeasure.'

Despite their extravagant character, it would be wrong to underestimate the possible effects – in some cases salutary – of such practices. For it is not inconceivable that, as a result of a psychological shock, previously repressed mechanisms would suddenly be released, and certain recoveries which were supposedly miraculous can be explained in this way.

One category of impotence recognised by the courts applied specifically to women, although experts in canon law took a long time to recognise the existence of female impotence. As late as 1610, when the dissolution of marriages for this reason was a well-established practice, one nevertheless finds Vincent Tagereau writing that a husband could lodge a suit against his wife if 'she be so narrow that she cannot be rendered large enough to have carnal relations with a man,' but adding that 'this almost never happens. And moreover, we do encounter no complaints on the part of husbands, but many on the part of wives.'

For several centuries, noted Esmein in 1891, 'canon law seems not to have taken account of this type of impotence, perhaps because in years gone by the conditions of everyday life made it difficult to conceal such anomalies, and marriage with a woman who was known to have such an incapacity was inconceivable.'

In the ninth century, the archbishop of Rheims, Hincmar, showed himself to be overtly hostile to separations based on such a pretext. Two centuries later, Pope Lucius III considered such unions to be impossible, and therefore impossible to dissolve. It was only under the pontificate of Innocent III

(1198–1216) that the chapter 'De Fraternitatis' institutionalised, under the title 'De Frigidis', the dissolution of marriages
for female impotence.

Trials for female impotence were, in fact, much rarer than
for male impotence. On the basis of an analysis of the few
dozen trials which have come down to us, the former would
seem to have constituted approximately five per cent of all
cases.

Like male impotence, female impotence could be natural or
accidental, curable or permanent, absolute or relative. As it
was linked to strictly physiological causes, it was less mysterious, less 'occult' than male impotence. Traditionally, a distinction was made between three types of sexual incapacity in
women.

The most frequent of these, in which the vagina is too narrow
to allow intromission, was referred to as 'arctitude'. The
second, and rarer, case was when a membrane of more or less
uniform consistency closed over the vagina. Finally, the neck of
the uterus could become blocked by a growth of flesh which
made all attempts at access impossible. The texts referred to the
latter malformation by the term *clausura*. Experts in forensic
medicine were careful to separate these three forms of impotence, for they did not all necessarily entail the dissolution
of the marriage bond.

'Arctitude', which meant unusual narrowness but not complete obstruction of the genital parts, made it impossible to
achieve coitus if the phallus was of unsuitable proportions. In
theory this form of impotence was perpetual, but in many cases
would prove to be only relative, and the marriage would
therefore remain valid, provided that the husband's member
was slightly smaller in diameter than the average.

In the second type, a membrane – which specialists termed a
velamen – blocked access to the vagina. It is important not to
confuse this with the more or less hypothetical film which

constitutes the hymen. According to Zacchia, however, the rigidity and thickness of some hymens occasionally present an obstacle which the most impetuous of male members cannot overcome. But in these cases it was necessary to identify such irregularities with *clausura*. The *velamen*, on the other hand, was sometimes finely textured, sometimes fleshy. It could be perforated or not, and depending on the individual case was located either in front of the external orifice, inside, or at the back of the vagina.

When it is 'delicate and finely tissued', it hardly interferes with intromission, and childbirth usually causes it to rupture. If it happens to be located at the back of the vagina coitus remains possible, but, to ensure that the woman should conceive, it was usual to perforate the *velamen* with small holes. 'In which case,' remarked Boucher d'Argis casually, 'the *velamen* does in no wise hinder the woman from conceiving, but does commonly cause her to die in childbirth.' This membrane came within the category of perpetual impotence, and when the appropriate authorities decided that an incision could not be performed, the marriage would be annulled. The success of such an operation depended upon a whole range of factors, and was easier and less offensive when the membrane was thin, fleshy and fibrous in texture, and when it was located near the external opening of the vagina, so as to be accessible to surgical instruments. Finally, it was essential that the patient should be young.

In the third type of female impotence, the neck of the womb is completely covered with fleshy growths which form a solid mass. According to Boucher d'Argis, this deformity could be either congenital or morbid in origin. 'If this condition be firmly developed and present from birth, it is incurable and does constitute a cause of perpetual impotence. If it be merely the result of an illness, and of recent date, it may easily heal of its own accord, in which case it has no power to annul the

marriage.' Sometimes a badly healed wound was the precipitating cause. Lazarus Rivierus even considered that this form of
clausura was always the after-effect of a wound or ulcer. In
such cases incision proved to be difficult, if not impossible.
Whether the membrane was composed of nerves or of flesh, the
husband was never allowed to decide upon an operation on his
own authority. The responsibility for such a decision rested
with the relevant experts, who alone were considered capable
of judging the consequences. On this point, the ruling of the
jurist Tomas Sanchez was categorical.

Apart from the three congenital malformations described
above, no other condition was recognised as making a woman
unable to perform coitus. Frigidity, which in the case of men
freezes the sexual parts into an inexplicable state of inactivity
and constitutes 'in the case of many husbands the reef upon
which their potency founders', was considered as having no
application to female sexuality. Certain wives, undeniably,
remained entirely numb to the caresses of their partners. No
matter, for this had no effect upon the functional aspects of
their sexual organs. As for sexual satisfaction – particularly in
women – it was regarded merely as a peripheral phenomenon.
Besides, it was not required of a woman that she achieve
orgasm; in fact the question was totally irrelevant. In the
opinion of Boucher d'Argis, the operations of the female
organism were mysterious, submerged. It was better to know
nothing about them than to accord an unnecessary importance
to a problem which was fundamentally insignificant. It was in
this spirit that Coquereau, writing in 1749, dismissed the
question of female frigidity: 'Frigidity in women does not
figure among the diriment impediments, for it is not possible to
examine what takes place internally, in those parts which are in
women the active parts.' The allusion to the passive role of the
wife during intercourse is here barely concealed. This notion
had already been formulated, a century and a half earlier, by

the Spaniard Tomas Sanchez: in the conjugal act, the woman plays an entirely passive role, and no contribution of passion is required of her, in contrast to the husband, whose role is active. Therefore, a disabling frigidity could not possibly exist in women. And the logical consequence of this belief was that female frigidity could not be construed as a diriment impediment in the same sense as a husband's failure to perform.

Jurists deliberately dissociated the sexual act from the notion of pleasure. As far as they were concerned, absolute conjugal perfection was achieved only when the three legal criteria of male virility were fulfilled: erection, intromission and emission. In the context of this reductive philosophy of marriage, female frigidity was of no interest, and jurists were entirely indifferent to the plight of those women who found it impossible to respond to the caresses of a brutish husband – provided that he functioned in accordance with the norms of Canon law. On the other hand, as we shall see, this indifference transformed itself into a frenzied eloquence when it came to feeling compassion for the fate of a woman whose husband happened to be impotent.

2

Ambiguous situations

Bordering upon impotence as such, there were a number of sexual and genetic irregularities which placed the individual in an ambiguous situation vis-à-vis the institution of marriage. Disorders of this kind proved difficult to integrate within the traditional forensic schema of impotence. Such things as marriages involving those who had not reached puberty, the elderly or the sterile became the object of discussions and controversies from which relatively coherent conclusions emerged. But the existence, let alone the marriages, of hermaphrodites raised far more difficult problems. It is true that such an extremely rare phenomenon did not arouse any impassioned controversy, and the debate which evolved around their equivocal nature was motivated chiefly by curiosity. Nevertheless, the solitary victims of such scrutiny faced a terrible reality.

The notion of hermaphroditism originated in a beautiful myth. The lyrical spirit of the ancient Greeks imagined the fruits of a union between Hermes and Aphrodite, called Hermaphroditus. Endowed with all the gifts of nature, his beauty seduced and troubled the nymph Salamis, who gave free rein to her desires one morning when she saw him bathing in the clear waters of a stream. However, maddened by his indifference, Salamis turned to the Gods, beseeching them to unite their two bodies in one. Her prayer was granted, but the sexual parts of the couple retained their separate identities without combining. Hermaphroditus in turn extracted the promise that, from then on, all who bathed in the waters of this stream would undergo the same transformation. And so the race of hermaphrodites was born.

Taking little heed of the poetic value of their myths, the Athenians and the Romans considered hermaphrodites to be monsters, and were accustomed to casting them into the sea and into the Tiber respectively. Yet, when the Romans discovered the existence of such prodigies of nature in the animal world, they 'used them for their pleasure', according to the jurist d'Arrerac. 'The first time that hermaphrodites were to be seen among four-footed animals, was during the Empire of Nero, who had a team of them to draw his coach: it being in keeping that the most fantastical man in the world should be drawn by such prodigies, the true symbol and mark of his monstrous and detestable life, and of the evils that accompanied his reign.' In the third century A D, the treatment of human hermaphrodites underwent a marked improvement, at the instigation of the jurisconsult Ulpien, who provided them with a relatively enlightened statute (*Lex Repetundarum*). Henceforth, they were to be regarded as either men or women, according to the sex which predominated in each case.

Throughout the Middle Ages and up until the sixteenth century, the situation of hermaphrodites seems to have been fairly ill-defined, and the stake was doubtless used on more than one occasion to sanction the anathema which hung over them as the children or henchmen of Satan. In some cases, moreover, they were probably buried alive. César de Rochefort's *Dictionnaire général et curieux* of 1685 records one such dreadful case: 'The year 1461, in a town in Scotland called L . . . , an hermaphrodite servant girl did get with child the daughter of her master. Being most rigorously pursued in justice for the reparation of this perfidious violation, she was condemned to be buried alive.'

From the beginning of the sixteenth century, the hermaphrodite found himself confined by a juridical structure which, although repressive in practice, was intended to be protective. Using the stipulations laid down in the *Lex Repetundarum* as his point of departure, the canon lawyer Sanchez resolved down to its finest details the difficult problem of the hermaphrodite's matrimonial status. Doctors and midwives were to be responsible for determining the sex which predominated in each case. According to their findings, the hermaphrodite was to be legally declared male or female in the fullest sense, and was entitled to marry a member of the opposite sex without prejudice. Where neither sex predominated, the hermaphrodite was allowed to choose, but having done so was legally bound to refrain from all use of the alternative sexual organs – an act which would constitute in the eyes of the Church a mortal sin and the crime of sodomy.

This legislation, which set the seal on this factitious social integration, could not dispel the persistent element of uncertainty which condemned the individual to a precarious social position. Clearly, the impulse to 'normalise' such ambiguities answered to a prior objective: to conform with a scientific point of view which no longer regarded sexual ambivalence as a monstrosity or an insult to God. But the canonists of the classical age, by a skilful and strategic sleight of hand, rejected the mediaeval version of the monstrous only to replace it by a dangerous moralising which served to incriminate all that was sexually equivocal. And in the case of hermaphrodites, this ethic of sexuality often proved deadly.

This insidious shift in values was to have tragic consequences. Several hermaphrodites, 'who,' wrote Brillon, 'having chosen the virile sex as the one that prevailed in them, subsequently behaved as women,' were condemned to the stake for the crime of sodomy. The verdict of the High Court of Paris in 1603, condemning one of these individuals to be hanged and then burnt at the stake, was by no means unique. By such means those who happened to be androgynous were forcefully prevented from exercising their dual sexuality as they pleased. Often unable to be classified as male or female, the hermaphrodite was readily accused of abominable vices – particularly when he or she was disposed towards a certain eclecticism of taste. And such accusations were not without an element of jealousy: 'It would indeed be indecent,' says Sanchez, 'were he entitled to use the one and then the other sex whenever he chooses.'

In spite of everything, it was not long before a more liberal attitude began to develop. Gradually, a scientific fact emerged from the farrago of myth and fantasy: that nature, by a subtle game whose rules were best known to herself, was able to conceal the sexuality of a woman behind the exterior of a man, and vice versa. However, 'this exterior, this skin, this semblance, does in no sense deceive the enlightened observer,' declared the *Grande Encyclopédie* by Diderot and D'Alembert in 1777. For some of these observers, the ambiguous nature of the hermaphrodite was an illusion. The extraordinary physical constitution of one Marin Le Marcis was offered as the tangible proof of this, and the misfortunes suffered by this unfortunate person might have been the catalyst for a new climate of opinion.

About the year 1581, in Monstiervillier, a modest village in the Caux region, a little girl was baptised under the name Marie Le Marcis. From the age of eight, she worked as a chambermaid in various houses of the region. Seven years later, she first began to experience the occasional movements of an intermittently present male organ, particularly in the presence of other women. The appearance of 'two fleshy growths or testicles below the penis, of the thickness of two acorns' gave the phenomenon a new dimension.

Presently a thirty-year-old widow, Jeane Le Febvre, entered the service of Marie's mistress, and the two chambermaids had to share the same bed. Marie's virile organ now extended itself once and for all, never to retract again. In the deposition of Jeane Le Febvre, we read that 'on divers occasions, when in bed, the said Marin did become excited and rage with desire for the aforementioned witness, though without ever revealing himself.' But it was not long before he yielded to temptation. One evening, when the two chambermaids were washing clothes, Marie informed her companion 'that she was in truth a boy and, upon showing her virile member, did ask the witness if she wished that they should marry together.' From then on, 'the witness would often touch and take in her hands the said virile member, which she realised to be indeed such, and of the same thickness or length as that of her late husband . . .' But Jeane Le Febvre also testified that although 'the said Marin did on divers occasions strive to enjoy the company of the witness, she did not wish to permit him, despite his vows and pledges to marry her.'

Shortly afterwards, however, we find Marie presenting Jeane to her parents, and announcing their intention to marry. Dumbfounded by all this, the parents endeavoured to 'distract' their daughter from 'the friendship of the said Le Febvre,' according to Marin Le Marcis, 'the more so that she was poor and without means, and that the widow had two children to support by her first husband.' At this point, Marie finally succeeded in achieving 'possession of the said Le Febvre, three or four times during the first night,' and thereafter on fourteen successive nights, 'not without repetition of the pleasant contest.'

Contented with their love-making, the future husband and wife sought out the elder of the village, who referred them to the Rouen penitentiary to obtain a dispensation to marry. Jeane and Marie set off. Upon arriving in Rouen, Marie changed her name to Marin and dressed for the first time as a man. The young couple presented themselves with a clear conscience at the penitentiary, where, to their astonishment, they were immediately arrested, imprisoned in the caretaker's lodge and handed over to the Court of Monstiervillier. The incarceration of Marin immediately brought about the nervous retraction of his male organ, and the experts were unanimous in denouncing what they regarded as trickery. In these circumstances, the affair took a sinister turn with the verdict of 4 May 1601:

Marie Le Marcis was duly charged and condemned for having unrightfully assumed the dress, usurped the name and attempted to counterfeit the sex of a man. And under this pretext to have committed with the said Jeane Le Febvre the crime of sodomy and abominable lustfulness. And, that she might the more freely abuse her said sex, of having essayed to hide this loathsome sin under the sacred cloak of marriage . . .

According to the summing up of the royal prosecutor:

Marie Le Marcis and Jeane Le Febvre are required and condemned to make honourable reparation with bare heads and bare feet . . . And afterwards, the said Marie Le Marcis is condemned to be burned alive, her body reduced to cinders, her chattels and inheritances acquired and confiscated by the King . . .

As for Jeane Le Febvre,

she is to be present at the execution of the said Marie Le Marcis, after which she is to be whipped and beaten with a birch on three successive market days, and banished from this province of Normandy, her chattels and inheritances acquired and confiscated by the King . . .

The King's prosecutor would have had Marin burned to death without any further form of trial, had not the unfortunate victim lodged an appeal with the High Court at Rouen. A second examination took place. Only one of the six experts, a surgeon by the name of Jacques Duval, courageously dared to 'probe the natural parts of the said Marin Le Marcis with his finger':

I placed my finger into the conduit of the said Marcis . . . What I did touch with the tip of my finger was a virile member, quite thick and hard . . . I could not rest satisfied until I had witnessed the said Marin, excited as he was by frequent stimulation, pour forth a white genital semen, thick and of normal fluidity.

It was thanks to Jacques Duval that Marin Le Marcis was saved from a terrible death. However, he was condemned to live as a woman, and so forced to content himself with a marginal social existence.

Indeed, it is impossible for a hermaphrodite to achieve any degree of real social integration. Despite a greater clemency on the part of judges, a deep-seated loathing still surrounded the figure of the hermaphrodite, and there were heavy penalties incurred for slandering somebody by even accusing him of being a hermaphrodite – especially if he happened to be an ecclesiastic. In one case the slanderer of a Canon was fined 300 livres, and the High Court of Toulouse further stipulated that the accused 'should demand pardon of the Canon on his knees before the prosecutor and at the door of the cathedral, in the presence of the chapter.' The purificatory aspect of this ritual gives some idea of the taint borne by the hermaphrodite.

Moreover, the status of hermaphrodites – which in theory was fixed – seems to have been determined in the most indecisive manner. Decisions as to the dominant sex in a particular case were slow. Malicious insinuations and slyly calculated contradictions placed the hermaphrodite in a situation which was often incriminatory and always tragic. One lengthy case illustrates this tendency.

In 1765 a strange memoir was published in Lyon, bearing the signature of Maître Vermeil. Its intention was to defend 'a certain individual who partook of the identity of both sexes, who was seen at divers times to wear the dress of a woman and a man, and who was baptised a girl but married as a boy.' The lawyer went on to state that this individual 'does today fasten the attention of magistrates and the curiosity of a public that is always avid for this kind of phenomenon.'

The story begins in 1732, when a child of apparently female sex was born in Grenoble and baptised under the name of Anne. In her fourteenth year, Anne Grandjean began to experience feelings whose nature astonished her. 'An instinct of pleasure, whose cause she did not know, unceasingly drew her to her female companions, and did develop in her a faculty which was in no sense appropriate to the sex to which at first she had been thought to belong. The presence of men, on the other hand, left her cold and unaffected.' Shortly afterwards, Anne Grandjean found herself equipped with all the attributes of masculinity. Her confessor was adamant that she could no longer dress as a girl without being in a state of grave sin. The news of her metamorphosis created a sensation and 'the young girls of the region looked upon her with a new interest.' At first, Grandjean was content to have a brief affair with one Legrand. Although this was a passing fancy of no apparent significance, it was later to have a considerable effect upon her destiny. Some years passed. 'He' now fell in love with one Françoise Lambert and married her. The publication of the banns did not occasion any opposition, and the marriage was celebrated in Chambéry on 24 June 1761.

There were no clouds to trouble the early years of married life. On the contrary, one new development lent an additional conviction to the role of man and husband which Grandjean had chosen. Françoise Lambert decided to give him a share in administering a family inheritance she had just come into. However, in a region where marriage did not confer independence, the young man was subject to paternal authority in such matters. He duly asked his father to grant him his independence, without which he could not embark upon any personal venture. This formality might have encountered an insuperable obstacle, for the parish register only referred to the existence of a girl named Anne Grandjean. However, the actual change of name and sex presented no difficulties. Henceforth, this new recruit to the male sex was to be known as Jean Baptiste, with nothing to interfere with his calm possession of this civil status. Or at least such was the assumption.

But it was at this point that, by a stroke of bad luck or malicious intention, Miss Legrand happened to become an intimate friend of Françoise Lambert and enlighten her as to the real nature of her husband. Perplexed, the young wife consulted her spiritual advisor, who ordered her to break off all familiarities with her husband. It was an insidious paradox, as Maître Vermeil noted in his memoir, that 'by a combination of circumstances each more remarkable than the other, it should have been a spiritual advisor who compelled Grandjean to take upon him the dress of a man, and a spiritual advisor who then compelled Françoise Lambert to deny her husband his identity as a man.'

Jean Baptiste wished to place the matter in the hands of the vicar-general. But the news of his predicament, obligingly spread about by Miss Legrand, was moving with lightning speed around a community which wallowed avidly in such subjects. Thus the deputy public prosecutor came to hear of the scandalous liaison which had for several years joined a female hermaphrodite and a woman. After an exhausting examination, Grandjean, who loudly protested his good faith as a man and husband, was placed under arrest and thrown into prison with his feet manacled. One painful circumstance of his arrest, in the light of which he seems an even more tragic figure, is that he could be incarcerated neither with men or women, as he was considered neither male nor female. Instead, he was placed in solitary confinement, in the dark of a narrow dungeon where he fed upon his misery in silence. Witnesses were questioned and the accused was visited. The report of his medical examination is a masterpiece of hypocrisy.

Inside the lips of the vagina the experts discovered a mass of flesh resembling a male organ. This growth, they said, became erect with excitement in the presence of a woman, and remained so during coitus. It was of the thickness of a finger while erect, and its length was equivalent to the width of four fingers across. At the tip of this male organ there was a glans with foreskin, but the glans was not perforated and could not emit any semen. Two testicles were apparent at the mouth of the vulva. The vulva itself was so narrow that a finger could be introduced into it only with difficulty. Menstruation did not occur and the vagina was not the source of any sensation of orgasm, nor did it emit any feminine sexual fluids.

Without any apparent relevance to the cause he was defending, Maître Vermeil's account revelled in an extraordinary profusion of details concerning the ambiguous physical constitution of his client:

Everything about him does appear to be a mixture of the two sexes in the same proportions of imperfectness . . . He is without beard, but has hairy legs. As to his breast, there is more of it than is customary in man, but it is in no sense delicate or sensitive to blows, unlike that of a woman: he did demonstrate this before us.

His nipples, if one is to consult their size, do belong to the female sex, but there is not to be found that circle of dark red in the centre which does characterise women.

His voice is, properly speaking, neither that of a woman nor of a man; rather it is that of a manchild who is approaching adolescence, and who, by a kind of huskiness, does make his sounds now deep, now shrill.

Grandjean was declared a female hermaphrodite. After a final interrogation, the court displayed an iniquitous, mediaeval severity towards him. He was condemned to wear an iron collar for three days, with an inscription around his neck bearing the motto 'Profaner of the Sacrament of Marriage', after which he was whipped and banished for life. And this was at the height of the Enlightenment.

Throughout this affair, the fundamental principles of canon law as they had been defined by Father Sanchez and reformulated, during the eighteenth century, by Le Semelier, were trampled underfoot. In reality, no structure or provision did exist to accommodate hermaphrodites. Tossed about according to the vague whims of each and everybody, Grandjean found himself successively baptised as a girl, dressed as a boy on the orders of one father confessor, but regarded as a usurper of the sacrament of marriage in the estimation of a second confessor. He was considered as a full citizen in the eyes of a regional administration, but condemned as an outrage to public decency on the orders of the royal administration. According to the report of the doctors he was neither male nor female, yet nevertheless guilty for having responded to the urgings of his deepest nature.

Even Maître Vermeil found himself compelled to acknowledge the crime and plead his client's good faith as a mitigating circumstance – a sad strategic retreat. The case was heard, and by a verdict of la Tournelle on 10 January 1765 Grandjean was acquitted of all charges of profanation, but ordered to revert to the dress of a woman and forbidden to 'haunt the company of Françoise Lambert and other persons of her sex.'

A deep social stigma thus weighed upon the hermaphrodite. In the same way as the impotent, and for the same reasons, he was consigned to the wretchedness of a marginal situation in society. Even in the most fortunate of circumstances he could be no more than an object of public curiosity and the victim of sordid exhibitions, as the surgeon B. Saviard recounts in 1702 in the case of Marguerite Malaure,

a native of Toulouse who arrived in Paris in the year 1693, in the guise of a boy, sword at his side, with his hair nonetheless hanging like that of a girl, and tied behind with a ribbon in the manner of the Spaniards and Neapolitans. She used to appear at public assemblies and allow herself to be examined for a small tip by those who were curious.

But Saviard smelt a rat, and Marguerite was taken to the Hotel-Dieu, where she became the object of an even more unwholesome demonstration:

I examined her [wrote Saviard] in each part with exactitude. I commenced with her breasts, that were very large like those of a woman of thirty years . . . I made her urinate before the gathered assembly, upon her claiming that her urine did issue from two separate places; and in order to make apparent the contrary, while she urinated I did spread apart the two lips of her vulva, by which means I did make the spectators see the urinary meatus from whence the flow did proceed exclusively . . .

Ultimately, it would seem that the fate of the ordinary impotent man or woman was more enviable than that of the hermaphrodite.

Another condition that constituted a diriment impediment to marriage was the absence or non-completion of puberty, and in the second chapter of *De Frigidis* those below the age of puberty are classified among the ranks of the impotent. In ancient Rome, where it was forbidden for citizens below the age of puberty to marry, the nubility of candidates for marriage was assessed in examinations of their genitals. But Justinian abolished this custom, which the Church considered to be obscene. From then on girls were recognised as pubescent at the age of twelve and boys at the age of fourteen. The Church's position was backed by moral and humanitarian reasons, as well as concern to ensure a rising birth rate.

The laws concerning puberty were made, according to the jurist Jean Papon, in the interests of the Republic and not

for such lecheries of youth as cannot yield any fruits other than imbecility [because] prior to the aforementioned age there cannot be engendered strong and robust men to assist the Republic through arms and service . . .

Moreover, young girls

being barely past the days when they sucked milk, and constrained by the labours of wedlock to serve as matrons and wives, are often stifled in the act of childbirth . . . others ofttimes do hanker lewdly to be with milk, or become incontinent after being enticed into this game . . .

As for over-youthful husbands, they are

enfeebled, and do remain lame, dissolute, are of short life or indeed of little service . . .

In the name of this utilitarian ethic, judges usually followed the letter of the law when handing out sentences. But the ban on marriages of the pre-pubescent does not seem to have been public law, and this type of union always received covert support if it was contracted with the consent of both families. 'It suffices that the spouses do persevere in their marriage and live together until full puberty of twelve years of age be accomplished,' wrote Brillon. However, this often resulted in ambiguous situations and misunderstandings. At the age of eleven, Françoise Frotier married Charles de la Tour. Eight months later, the marriage was legally ratified. At the age of twenty-three, the young woman requested an annulment and cited the circumstances in which the marriage had been contracted. The case was judged on appeal by the criminal court of la Tournelle, and Françoise Frotier was 'condemned to return to her husband.'

This type of 'prohibited' marital union was occasionally revealed, in dramatic circumstances, by the death of a pre-pubescent wife. Often it was only at this point that the parents of the unfortunate girl would realise that the marriage had not been valid and that there was still time to recuperate the dowry. One ten-year-old girl died six weeks after the marriage celebrations. The husband appropriated her possessions, but the sister of the deceased opposed this and brought the case before the High Court of Rouen. The verdict of 15 June 1655 ruled that 'all movables shall be returned to the uterine sister, less 1500 livres for the funeral expenses paid by the husband.'

Ultimately there was nothing to prevent the marriage of those below the age of puberty, provided that nobody opposed it. The jurist Soefve implicitly admitted this when he wrote concerning one marriage in which both partners had been pre-pubescent: 'This so-called marriage took place without any state of financial need or family consideration, though such are ofttimes the reasons for which such marriages are countenanced.'

The fundamental question is whether we should equate pre-pubescence with impotence. Did the established order feel itself threatened by such marriages? This seems unlikely, since a pre-pubescent individual did not violate the laws of nature. He or she was neither a monster nor a marginal within society in the same sense as a eunuch or a hermaphrodite. The canonical prohibition of marriages between the pre-pubescent reflected strictly moral considerations. For this reason the prohibition was not strong enough to counter powerful family or political reasons for contracting these unions.

It was possible, in spite of everything, to preserve a good conscience by waiting until puberty before marrying off partners who had been betrothed from the age of eight years. 'At this age,' points out Soefve, 'which is at bottom the age of reason, we do assume that the pre-pubescent have advanced sufficiently in judgement to be cognizant of their actions.'

As good logicians, the theologians and jurists of the classical period inevitably included the marriage of the elderly within the same category of condemnation that applied to the impotent. 'Dotage,' stated Boucher d'Argis, 'is oft accompanied by infirmities that may render one incapable of generation, and, if all old men be not disabled, it is certain, at least, that they do lack the fire and vigour of the young. That is why certain authors do seem to accuse them of that defect of frigidity which does extinguish in man all the desires and motions that do bend to the propagation of his species.'

There is a long history to the notion of old age as a kind of illness. It is reported that Diogenes called it *vitae brumatis* (the winter of life) and Cicero *vitae occasus* (the twilight of life). Saint Jerome regarded old men as ill. The theologian Fevret stated that the aged 'ought to be judged unfit to enter into wedlock ... The cold winter of their late season has extinguished all natural vigour, and the blood, half-frozen in their veins, is no longer capable of heat.' Zacchia compared old men to eunuchs and roundly declared that the wife of a septuagenarian could safely be counted among the ranks of the widowed.

It was therefore not without reason that the Romans, in accordance with the law *Pappia Poppeia*, forbade any man over the age of sixty to marry a woman below the age of fifty, and any woman over the age of fifty to marry a man below the age of sixty. This step was taken primarily in the interests of a rising birth rate. In the course of the wedding ceremony, the partners had to declare publicly that they were uniting in marriage in order to produce a lineage.

However, the early Christians prided themselves upon having a more elevated conception of conjugal relations. For them, procreation was merely one aspect of marriage, and, as early as the sixth century, Justinian repealed the *Pappia Poppeia* law.

There were several arguments in favour of marriage between the elderly. Boucher d'Argis expounded these with conviction. It was difficult, he wrote, to specify a strict age-limit beyond which an individual could be deemed unsuitable for procreation. Biblical history teaches us that Zacchary and Elizabeth were both advanced in age when the latter gave birth to Saint John the Baptist. Other examples were a certain Numidian king, who became a father at the age of eighty, or Cato the Censor, at the age of eighty-eight, or Vladislas of Poland, at the age of ninety.

Moreover, theologians were very careful to distinguish between 'fecundity' and the 'capacity to fulfil the conjugal duties.' Some old men might well be beyond the stage of procreating, but remained nonetheless capable of normal sexual relations. According to Boucher d'Argis, 'there is no age that may be considered as the absolute term of potency and the certain season of entire frigidity.' 'Besides,' he adds, not without a trace of hypocrisy, 'were it a constant and recognised fact that the aged persons that do come forward for marriage were entirely impotent, it is to be believed that the Church would in no sense administer the sacrament to them.'

In fact, the validity of marriage between the elderly was largely dependent upon a view of Christian charity. The Church regarded marriage as a social and charitable bond by which the partners were obliged to give each other mutual help and comfort. If anything, this bond was the stronger when it united the elderly with those who were somewhat younger, for the former 'are in far greater need of it than are the latter,' and because 'the inconveniences there would be in excluding the aged from the sacrament would far outweigh those that might result from the cohabitation of youth with a decrepit and frozen dotard.'

But not all jurists accepted without qualification the arguments of Boucher d'Argis on the principle of elderly marriages. Instead they drew attention to the fact that old age is primarily synonymous with impotence.

In spite of this, impotence trials had in fact little chance of success when the accused was of an advanced age. Arguments which would lead to marital disintegration for a young couple tended to work in favour of an old man.

A certain Magdeleine Pigousse married an old and impotent man. When she instigated legal proceedings against him, the result was to bring down upon herself the wrath of the assistant public prosecutor, Lamoignon, who attacked her in front of the entire assembled High Court of Paris:

It is only to herself that she may attribute her misfortune. For she ought to have been prepared when she did marry this ancient gentleman, de Saint Rémy, aged sixty-five years. A girl deceived by fine appearances, and by the flowering of youth that she did behold in her future husband . . . such a girl, I repeat, has some reason to complain before the judges, concerning the error into which she has been deceived, and to request the dissolution of her marriage bond. But what can this Mademoiselle Pigousse have hoped of a husband of sixty-five years?

The case of Magdeleine Pigousse is revealing. The elderly were permitted to marry inasmuch as their virility was granted the benefit of the doubt and their age the benefit of charity. In this context, complaining wives were always regarded with suspicion. But only when one considers the frequency of marriages of convenience during the *Ancien Régime* and the age disparity of couples united in this manner, is it possible to gain some idea of the miseries endured by very young women. But of course, it did not matter if a young wife had to submit to 'tortures of the flesh', provided that she sacrificed herself for the satisfaction of an old man.

Ultimately, a one-sided notion of charity was enshrined in the logic of the system. Verdicts of exclusion were freely pronounced upon the impotent, because this fundamentally egocentric practice was in a sense reassuring. It facilitated the assertion of one's own conformity to the established norms. But, by the same token, the jurists of the classical period were unable to place old age in the category of impotence without sooner or later including themselves, as a matter of course, within the 'structures of exclusion' which they had themselves fashioned.

Unlike the Greeks and Romans, Christians did not regard sterility as a reason for the annulment of marriage. There was a noble precedent for this: the marriage of Joseph and Mary was no less valid for being sterile. Thus, in spite of the evangelical imperative 'Be fruitful, and multiply, and replenish the earth' (Genesis IX, 1), procreation, as distinct from sexual inter-course, was never presented as a canonical necessity. The sacrament of marriage was instituted by God in order to counteract fornication as much as to ensure the propagation of the species, and its purpose was fulfilled by the accomplishment of either of these two functions. Besides, no individual could be held accountable for a sterility which came from the workings of the divine will. The jurist Sébastien Roulliard wrote, 'Man and woman are indeed the instruments of generation, but it is God who by his blessing produces the fruit.' Other writers repeated the same beliefs during the seventeenth and eighteenth centuries.

Some commentators went further than this, and the surgeon Guillemeau courted heresy when he asserted that 'the generation of children for posterity is but an accessory and frivolous dependancy of marriage, not the best part, and therefore in no sense a necessary aspect of the institution, as it is not required for the preservation of mankind that all men should engender offspring.'

In actual fact, this point of view was qualified by a severe religious restriction. The Church forbade all sexual activity undertaken in a spirit of pleasure for its own sake. The hope or ulterior motive of conception had always to be present during the conjugal act, according to St Augustine. This ambiguity was reflected in the impotence trials, where sexual relations were presented above all as a cure for sinful lust, but where the imperative of procreation was not, however, excluded from the proceedings. The canonical justification for such proceedings was even founded upon the procreative argument. When the early Church, in exceptional cases, allowed the annulment of a marriage on the grounds of impotence, any woman who felt starved of conjugal caresses could turn to her bishop and say, in the words of a traditional formula, 'I wish to become a mother, I wish to bear children, and to this end I have taken a husband; but the man whom I chose is frigid by nature and cannot provide what I expect of him.'

The importance accorded to procreation in the medical examination reports is also revealing. Before being judged impotent, the accused who were examined were portrayed primarily as 'incapable of procreation'. 'He could achieve no intromission into the usual vessel,' reads one report, 'so that the semen was spilt outside and consequently, procreation could not ensue.'

It would also seem that sterility was accepted as a reason for the dissolution of marriage bonds in princely houses, according to the canon lawyer Choppin, although he was refuted by Le Semelier. Choppin reports that the divorce of Louis XII and Jeanne de France was because of sterility: 'The sterility of one of the spouses in a marriage has been deemed legitimate cause, principally amongst the French, for the dissolution of the marriage bond.' But this did not apply to the common run of people. Concerning the latter, one case, which was judged on appeal on 13 April 1649, is often invoked. 'It is said,' specifies the verdict, 'that a wife may not have her husband cited, in order to effect the dissolution of the marriage contracted between them, on the grounds of her claiming that his seed be not prolific and that he is unable to engender.'

In reality, because of its pretensions to channel the sexual drives of the faithful, the Church was somewhat reluctant to impugn the conjugal act as such. It modestly took refuge behind the noble necessities of procreation. At the same time, in paradoxical fashion, the Church absolved those afflicted with sterility only to lay all blame upon the impotent – a phallocentric reaction, behind which loomed the visions of horror conjured up by the marriage of those afflicted by frigidity.

3

The problem of marriage

By marrying, the impotent man commits an act of larceny, profanes a sacrament, and indulges in an inhumane, cruel and dangerous act. These were the three themes which, from the beginning of the sixteenth century to the end of the eighteenth century, recurred incessantly in the writings of jurists and theologians.

In effect, these formulations depended upon a new and paradoxical conception of marriage. Theologians had elevated this institution to the heights of a sacrament, whereas from the end of the sixteenth century jurists had reduced it to the level of a common transaction. It became a 'synallagmatic' [reciprocal] contract (Boucher) or a 'redhibitory' [revocable] act (Peleus), in the spirit of which 'the Burgundians and Saxons had been accustomed to purchasing their wives from parents and guardians.' Anne Robert, in 1627, regarded marriage as no more than a 'form of sale or purchase transaction', which is why 'grievances are to be expected if one party holds back some secret wilfully and silently . . . Just as in the market place, the buyer should be assured against any vice or secret defect that might be hidden in the thing sold.' From this kind of analogy came the accusation of 'stelionnat' [fraud] which weighed over the impotent, who, in the words of Anne Robert, dared to 'enlist themselves in the holy and sacred militia of legitimate love, without possessing those dotal weapons that are necessary to the accomplishment of the wedding solemnities.' Moreover, 'if frauds and trickeries should be punished by the taint of infamy and dishonour, then in the case of marriage they are punishable by and do merit a torture worthy of our disapprobation.'

Like Anne Robert, the Toulouse lawyer D'Arrerac was among the first to popularise the notion of fraud in matters of impotence. 'The impotent,' he wrote,

> are mockers and affronters who have committed the crime of *stelionnat*, having passed off false wares for true, and having committed an imposture. That village girl, who was condemned not long since to be whipped for assuming the guise of a man and marrying the daughter of her master of whom she had become enamoured, did no more deserve this penalty than do these imposters.

The dissemination of this idea among the common people is attested by the existence of a broadsheet which repeated D'Arrerac's text word for word. Moreover, all legal works up until the end of the eighteenth century referred to the text.

The opinion expressed by Gayot de Pitival in 1743 was even more severe. After invoking, like the others, the authority of D'Arrerac, he proceeded to compare the impotent with counterfeiters 'that do contaminate all commerce with a coin of doubtful quality; they deceive not only the women whom they do wed, but the parents who do entrust them with their daughters.' And this false coin, so the argument runs, is all the more dangerous in that it creeps surreptitiously into the commerce of the flesh. 'Is there any man,' he continues, 'to whose snares we are more vulnerable? For beneath the finest appearances in the world, an impotent man does merely seduce a girl by contracting marriage with her.'

And how could one fail to pity the unfortunate victim who, seduced by hollow appearances, discovers in her marriage bed that she has taken a mere shadow for a husband? Consequently, she was entitled to claim damages. This step was all the more justified in that she would subsequently find that her value on the marriage market had depreciated. It was in fact 'rare that a man should desire to marry a woman whom a judge had separated from her husband on the grounds of the latter's impotence,' according to Le Semelier.

Far from any such venal considerations, the Fathers of the Church had elevated marriage to the status of a sacrament. By marrying, the impotent man deliberately violated this sacrament and, according to Gayot de Pitival, committed 'an attack upon the authority of the Church.' For Peleus, the insolent individual who acted under such false pretences was 'shameless in violating and prostituting marriage, which is the holiest and most sacred thing beneath the heavens.' The Abbé Le Semelier condemned such unions which, in his eyes, were nothing more than 'an insult to the sacrament and a profanation of its sanctity.' The marriage of an impotent was a 'mortal sin', a 'sacrilege'. This profanation was regarded as all the more contemptible since a savage prejudice commonly imputed to the impotent man an unbridled lasciviousness, exposing him to 'hidden vices that are forbidden to Christians.' For more than three centuries, these unfortunate individuals were treated with pious abjection. They were seen as

embracing in strange positions, indulging in illicit loves, and committing the crime of impiousness by defiling the nuptial bed through forbidden acts of sexual union. What horrors do they not inspire in a religion as pure as ours, since they use the veil of the sacrament to indulge in a commerce that is sullied with the most shameful prostitutions.

The impossibility of satisfying their desires, far from deadening these, does serve only to inflame them the more.

[For] all such immodest embraces between husband and wife, that bear no relation to normal usages of marriage, are sinful.

Not content with committing an outrage against religion, impotent men were now seen as sacrificing the happiness of their wives to the demands of their own lasciviousness, and the wives were often portrayed as pathetic victims suffering a martyrdom of physical deprivation.

The sexual function of marriage was generally regarded and

tolerated as the least offensive way of accommodating the unhealthy demands of the flesh. In the opinion of Anne Robert, 'women do suffer more the stings of desire for these pleasures than do men, and cannot, in their infirmity, so easily forego them.' The doctor allows the patient to drink, not to cure him of his fever, but to help him endure it better. Using this comparison, Anne Robert drew attention to the fact that virginity or chastity was a state of perfection attainable only by the few. The rest of us find in marriage an adequate panacea, whereby 'through pleasure and mutual ardour, the fleshly desires of youth are abated.'

The wife of an impotent man is therefore, by analogy, an invalid deprived of treatment. As far as D'Arrerac was concerned, 'a husband that is emasculate, cold, languid, frozen to the marrow, and who can do nought of what he has promised his wife, is the very quintessence of misfortune' and represents moreover a mortal danger. The story of Eusebia, the wife of the emperor Constantine, was considered a sad illustration of this fact. She died 'in the flower of youth, consumed by the passion natural to her age, . . . for want of the pleasing sweetness of conjugal union.'

A breath of pathos rises from the prose of Anne Robert when he laments the fate of a young wife brutally confronted with the fact of her husband's impotence:

Never shall I be persuaded that a new bride should derive pleasure from lying with a husband who, after the festivities and solemnities of a perfect wedding, and during the first embraces – accompanied by strong caresses though without ever coming to the principal point of the operation – does set to discoursing in praise of virginity, and who, colder than all ice, does become heated in philosophising on chastity.

In none of the impotence trials did the plaintiff refrain from complacently parading the sufferings associated with her pitiable condition. It was always the same testimony, the same cry of distress. Frustrated and defenceless, tormented by desire, flayed alive by her sexual urges, she was forced in addition to face the crazed assaults of a husband whose impotence had made him wild and who attempted to divest her of her virginity by the most unorthodox means.

Before the magistrates of the High Court of Aix-en-Provence, Suzanne Auguier threw all discretion to the winds in describing the behaviour of her husband, Henri Fermier, who 'would pass entire nights upon her body, forcing her to suffer inconceivable distress and pain, and, after a thousand vain efforts, employing his fists and hands rather than those natural parts that were incapable of erection, would finally leave her in the same state as he had found her on the first night that he did enter the nuptial bed.'

Other testimonies reveal similarly apocalyptic scenes. De Bray and De Langey were described as employing 'iron fitments' to crack the virginity of their wives. The dangers to which Suzanne de Machy was exposed were used as the main argument by her lawyer, Maître Severt, in the trial against Jacques François Michel. According to Severt,

Truly, it were to expose Modesty to hazardous and criminal excesses, were we to let a wife remain prey to the abominations and infamies with which she is contaminated in the company of a counterfeit husband. If he be allowed to satisfy with impunity his brutish furies, this were to kindle in his wretched victim, by a multitude of unnatural vices, a pernicious and unceasing flame that it would be impossible to extinguish by any legitimate means, short of recourse to the salutary remedy of the conjugal duty itself.

A similar sentiment prompted Maître Begon, the lawyer of Marie Magdeleine Mascranni, the frustrated wife of the Marquis de Gesvre:

You are uncognisant of the cruel assaults that she is forced to endure, and of what a trial it is that the image of a husband devoid of substance should yet be able to kindle in her those dark flames which burn only to defile. What can I say of the perils that do threaten her modesty, and of the continual alarms to which her life is exposed? We know to what extremes the fury of an impotent husband is capable of leading him, when he feels that Nature does flee his exertions . . .

Some husbands were even prepared to place matters in the hands of other men in the attempt to give their marriages the seal of legitimacy:

It is also known that, following the example of a certain king of Castille, these counterfeit husbands do try to cleanse their shame in the crime of another; that they purchase honour by passing for fathers, to which end they sacrifice the honour of the nuptial bed, and that they turn into pandars for those to whom they are unable to be husbands. The king was not alone who rendered himself guilty of this infamous policy; many of his fellow impotents have imitated him.

Another king, Don Alphonse of Portugal, was reputed to have installed a secret door in the queen's bedroom, close to the bed curtains, so that someone from outside could come and go unobserved by anyone else in the room. In the High Court of Paris, the case against Jean Auffroy contained this accusation:

. . . that he did say to her [his wife] that if she desired to have children, as he knew that she did like them greatly, she might invite to herself someone; that he would not find it amiss, that on the contrary he would be well pleased to have a child.

Finally, the marriage of the impotent man even becomes impregnated with the odour of death:

The wife of the impotent is a living body narrowly confined with a dead body. For, just as death may not take carnal possession of a living body, because the dead are incapable of enjoying a woman, in like manner the impotent husband is unable to possess the body of his wife . . . As all that may in the end result from the union of a dead body with a living body is to make the living body fall into rottenness; so all that may proceed from the union of a woman with an impotent is to make her contaminate.

All means were valid, therefore, to discredit an impotent man, so as to exclude him from a society upon whose civil and religious order his existence had a disruptive effect. Marriage, evidently, was forbidden him. On the other hand, when a woman, duly informed as to the impotence of her betrothed, wished in spite of everything to marry him and live as sister and brother, was there any valid reason for preventing her?

The reply to this question was ambiguously formulated, and placed the theologians of the classical period in a contradictory position to that of their mediaeval predecessors. For the decrees and canons of the Church were categorical: the fraternal cohabitation of husband and wife represented an elevated conception of marriage based on chastity and the intimate union of two souls.

Until the thirteenth century, Popes therefore advised impotent husbands to live as brothers with their wives. However, from the twelfth century, the Gallican Church appears to have admitted the principle of marriage annulments in cases of impotence, and when Gregory IX (1227–41) set about codifying Canon law, he aligned himself with the latter position.

This departure ended in an astonishing and unlawful decision by Celestin IV, who became Pope in 1241. This decree allowed a husband, whose wife's sex was too narrow, both to keep her in his house and to remarry. However, history has not preserved any evidence as to the implementation of a decree which effectively ratified bigamy. Equally, we do not know what would have been the reaction of the Holy Father to a wife requesting the same privilege.

In spite of everything, fraternal cohabitation, which was constantly exalted, remained the image of an ideal perfection. The appeal for an annulment on the grounds of impotence was regarded as a last resort, and granted only when sexual continence proved impossible for the other partner. But the great canonical reaction which took place during the sixteenth century – already illustrated in the hostility of Sixtus V towards eunuchs – could not afford to tolerate such liberal attitudes. It soon became a matter of the greatest urgency to reverse the status of impotence, which, far from confining the individual within rigid structures of exclusion, made him into a kind of model of evangelical purity.

The problem remained as to how to formulate points of view which would quite clearly place the theologians in flagrant contradiction to the spirit and the letter of Canon law. It was necessary to play on words, to juggle with language. Undeniably, conjugal chastity did represent an ideal state. But the Popes, aware of the demands of sexuality, could only 'recommend' this ideal. 'It is to be preferred . . .', 'The Church counsels . . .' are the phrases which crop up in the decrees (*bonum esset, consuetudo est Romanae ecclesiae, Ecclesia consuevit . . .*).

So restrictive an interpretation of the words of the early Popes was clearly made with the intention of misrepresenting them. For the theorists of the classical period, the 'counsel' and advocacy of chastity drew its inspiration from an excessively refined conception of human nature. Sexual continence in marriage was merely a fiction, an abstraction. In reality – which was rather more prosaic – the wife of an impotent man was prey to the lascivious excesses and perverse wit of a spirit unhinged by its disability. By the same token, a 'narrow' wife incited her husband to immodest caresses and perilous sexual deviations. This line of argument was clearly formulated, as early as the beginning of the sixteenth century, by Father Sanchez.

By the eighteenth century, Bouhier could remark that 'it is commonly acknowledged that nothing is more difficult than to persuade impotents to relinquish conjugal love for brotherly companionship.' Again, Le Semelier describes, in derisive tones, how impotent husbands 'must sign a pact with each of their senses, suppress everything that might in any way allow friendship to degenerate into passion, preserve their corporeal vessel in innocence and honour, and resist following the dissolute promptings of concupiscence.' The author goes on to observe that this presupposes a degree of self-control and self-denial of which nobody is in fact capable. The implicit rejection of pontifical rulings about fraternal cohabitation follows from this imperturbable logic.

At this level, the impotent individual was the object of systematic attempts to exclude him categorically from the matrimonial sacrament. But the question remained as to whether there existed a temporal authority with the power to prevent the marriage of a couple who were aware of the disability which weighed over them and nevertheless wished to marry.

The application of the canonical interdicts was complicated by a considerable practical difficulty: the detection of conjugal incapacity. Four different types of detection had to be considered.

Sometimes the impotent partner was denounced by a third party opposed to the marriage, sometimes by a well-informed parish priest who would refuse to publish the banns. Alternatively, the fiancée, warned in time about her partner's disability, could obtain from the ecclesiastical judge an interdiction forbidding the marriage to be held. Finally, there were cases where the future husband would publicly reveal his own impotence and, by the same token, terminate the engagement. The interdiction on a particular marriage would depend upon the specific conditions under which it was denounced. What form did these take for each of the above categories?

The presumed impotent was denounced by a third party, usually a relative who disapproved of the marriage. This intervention was nearly always motivated by sordid financial considerations. In theory, it had little chance of success.

Thus in 1639 an inhabitant of Pamiers decided to get married. His brother tried to prevent him, on the grounds that he lacked 'those natural parts necessary for marriage.' The accused retorted that 'the beauty, whom the matter most concerned, had no complaints, and, when this was no longer the case, she would have him *tamquam patrem, non tanquam maritum*' (as a father if not as a spouse). The parliament of Toulouse ruled that the marriage could proceed. Needless to say, 'the beauty' had been made heiress to a tidy little fortune.

In 1655, a man from Caudebec in Normandy contested the marriage of his uncle, a certain De La Mare. The latter was a widower, but without any children. Before the local judge, the impetuous nephew claimed that his uncle was impotent. He sought to prove this 'by the mere inspection of his outward appearance: he is without hairs and he has the face of an impotent.' Receptive to this line of argument, the judge returned a verdict which was favourable to the nephew's wishes. But De La Mare brought the case on appeal before the High Court at Rouen. Such an accusation, he claimed, could be made only by his wife. Moreover, the young man had betrayed his real motives by accusing the uncle of wishing to disinherit him. The verdict of the Caudebec judge was quashed and De La Mare finally received permission to marry.

On the other hand, the same accusation made by a parish priest concerning a member of his flock would involve quite different considerations. In 1655, a verdict of the High Court of Paris had immense repercussions for the procedures concerning detection and denunciation.

Denis Pinot, a native of Le Mans, was about to marry Marie Bulot. Parental consent had been given and a marriage contract drawn up in due form, in the presence of a notary. The couple requested the publication of the banns, whereupon they met with a categorical refusal from the parish priest 'on the grounds that, by common knowledge, Denis Pinot was considered to be a eunuch.' The unfortunate man served a writ upon the priest, charging him to appear before the lieutenant general, who eventually ordered the accused to state whether he was in fact impotent. Upon receiving an affirmative answer, the court confirmed the priest's decision not to publish the marriage banns. However, the betrothed couple now lodged an appeal to the High Court of Paris.

The case was heard on 8 January 1665 'in audience of the great chamber', before which Denis Pinot and Marie Bulot maintained that their parish priest had encroached upon the prerogatives of the family, and that the admission of impotence had been extorted by unfair means. Besides, Marie and her family had not been kept in ignorance of the truth. Therefore there was nothing to stand in the way of the wedding celebrations.

The parish priest of Le Mans pointed out that, on the contrary, Pinot's impotence was 'commonly acknowledged' and that he could not grant his request without gravely abusing the holy sacrament. But the assistant public prosecutor, Talon, argued in favour of the young couple, and pointed out that there was something distinctly odd about the priest's behaviour. For, if he was informed as to the impotence of a member of his flock through the confessional, he could not reveal such knowledge without committing a crime. If, on the other hand, public gossip had brought this supposed impotence to his attention, surely modesty ought to prevent him from speaking of it.

In spite of this eloquent plea, the court rejected the appeal and the litigants were ordered to pay the costs of the hearings.

The opinion of a fiancée as to the impotence of her future husband seems also to have had every likelihood of being taken seriously, leading in certain cases to the breaking off of an engagement.

On 5 January 1607, the High Court of Paris returned a verdict in favour of Claudine Godefroy, 'that there were sufficient grounds for her not to proceed with the celebration of marriage with the man to whom she was betrothed.' It is worth noting the entirely iniquitous character of this verdict. The doctors and surgeons responsible for examining the genitals of the future husband had found that he had only a single testicle, which, they specified, did not in any way compromise his procreative faculties.

In cases where a man revealed his impotence of his own accord and asked that his engagement be ended, there were often grounds for suspecting him of using impotence as a last resort to extricate himself from an impossible situation.

On 26 May 1662, at the age of seventy, Nicholas Le Pot celebrated his engagement to Catherine Le Lectier, forty years his junior. According to the terms of the marriage contract, Catherine was to be housed and fed, and would have at her disposal a chambermaid, a valet, and a life income of 500 livres. On 29 May, the marriage banns were published in the parish of Saint-Paul and Saint-Gervais. The marriage was planned for 1 June. In the meantime, however, Le Pot began to have second thoughts, changed his mind about the wedding, and decided that he was impotent. On the wedding day, there was no husband in sight. His conscience troubled, he had gone to the Sorbonne instead of presenting himself at the church. There, he sought the advice of four doctors of divinity. He set forth his case and requested them to provide him with a written opinion. His fate decided, he then returned to the place where the wedding celebrations were to be held. There he presented his fiancée with a brief letter specifying that

1. His impotency being perpetual, his marriage would be null and he would sin in contracting it.
2. To contract the said marriage on the condition of living together as brother and sister, would be to deceive the Church and abuse the sacraments.
3. When questioned by the priest as to whether he knew of any impediment to the marriage that he was about to contract, he would commit perjury were he to say no.

The ecclesiastical judge to whom the case was referred declared the marriage promise 'null and void', and invited Catherine Le Lectier to lodge an appeal with the relevant authorities for a settlement of the costs of litigation and to reclaim damages.

In fact, the interdiction placed upon those who were impotent does not appear to have constituted an insurmountable obstacle where both partners, fully informed as to their situation, decided nevertheless to proceed with the marriage. The ease with which the prohibition was infringed, even by those who were subject to an earlier verdict of annulment, is proof of this, and the notoriety of the verdict against Pinot indicates that it was an exception to the rule. The repressive apparatus set up by theologians and jurists during the seventeenth century thus exhibited one major flaw: it was powerless to act against partners who colluded. However, this was only one of the complex problems raised within the framework of these legal and forensic procedures for marital annulment.

4

The impotence trial in context

In canon law, impotence was a diriment impediment to marriage when it existed prior to the wedding ceremony. However, the procedures for annulment on these grounds did not become established in the ecclesiastical courts without some difficulty.

Originally, Roman laws were unaware of the effects of impotence upon marriage. It is true that the liberal practice of divorce always made it possible discreetly to terminate non-consummated unions. But the specific provision for separations on the grounds of impotence only became necessary when, during the Late Empire, Justinian began to censure divorce with civil penalties. Thus it was a charter of Justinian – cited endlessly by commentators during the classical period – which first recognised the legitimacy of divorce in cases where the marriage had not been consummated after two years of cohabitation. This probationary period was moreover increased from two to three years by a subsequent charter of Justinian.

The matrimonial system in Teutonic church law ruled out any possibility of taking legal action in cases of impotence. Divorce by mutual consent was permitted, but the right of repudiation was restricted to the husband, which limited the possibilities for the wife of an impotent man.

The western Church naturally opposed on principle the Germanic custom, whose influence it was endeavouring to check. It is clear that, at first, pontifical rulings encouraged fraternal cohabitation, while the Holy See would receive only with extreme reluctance appeals based on the impotence of one partner.

Around the same period, the ideological stance of the Gallican Church was more or less identical. In fact, Hincmar, the archbishop of Rheims, deemed that separations based on the pretext of impotence fermented discord and endangered the sacrament of marriage.

In reality, however, the synodal rulings and Carolingian collections of ordinances were adopting a quite new standpoint with regard to impotence. Towards the middle of the eighth century, the Council of Verberie restored her freedom to any wife who could prove the impotence of her husband by the ordeal of the cross. Again, the Council of Compiègne in 757 recognised separation on the grounds of impotence, on condition that the husband did not protest his virility, 'for he is master of the wife'.

The same stipulations were repeated in 827, in the fifty-fifth capitulary of the sixth book of the collection of Anségise. But it was still the task of the wife to furnish proof of her husband's impotence.

When the principle of marital indissolubility became established, it was essential to provide annulment procedures with a solid canonical justification. Hincmar of Rheims seems to have been the first to attempt a legal rationale. According to him, the Church fathers taught that marriage acquires the status of a sacrament only if it is validated by the union of the flesh. Impotence which exists at the time of the nuptial celebrations should therefore be considered as a legitimate motive for dissolving the marriage, and the wife should be entitled to provide for herself elsewhere on the grounds of sexual incontinence.

But it was the triumph of the principles of the Gallican Church which provided the annulment procedures with new canonical foundations. According to Peter Lombard, marriage became ratified as a sacrament from the moment that the vows were exchanged. In the case of impotence, there were two possible solutions: to confirm the validity of the sacrament by advising fraternal cohabitation, in accordance with the decrees of the Church, or to charge the impotent partner with matrimonial incapacity by declaring the marriage null and void. On this point the Gallican Church was to dissociate itself from the Roman Church, by promulgating the principle of annulment which, a few centuries later, the theologians of the classical period were to impose on the whole of Christianity.

It was only under the pontificate of Gregory IX (1227–41) that the Roman Church aligned itself with the Gallican Church on this matter, and that the decrees inserted under the heading *De Frigidis et Maleficiatis* made impotence a diriment impediment in the strict sense of the term. Moreover, it is likely that, for several more centuries, the application of this new doctrine was quite limited. Certainly, the legal apparatus was in place from the fifteenth century, since the departmental archives of the Aube region report the case of an 'impotent' whose marriage was dissolved in 1426, and who went on to have several children by his second wife. But the golden age of the impotence trial did not really begin until the sixteenth century.

At the same time as these developments, the system of evidence used in the proceedings also evolved appreciably. Originally, when a wife declared an unfulfilled desire to bear children, she had to provide proof of her husband's impotence by calling upon the testimony of seven relatives, friends or neighbours – this was known as proof by *septima manus*. The Roman Church was satisfied with this degree of intervention, which it regarded as sufficient to justify the dissolution of a marriage.

The Gallican Church would perhaps have relied exclusively upon the husband's assertion (*quia caput est mulieris*) had not certain aspects of Germanic practice filtered into the procedures for marital separation. Although ordeals by fire or by boiling water are sometimes referred to, it appears that trial by the cross was most frequently employed. The rulings of the Council of Verberie in 752 and the decree of Yves de Chartres in the eleventh century mention the latter as a standard procedure. Jurists of the classical period were divided as to the form which this ordeal took. Some believed that the champions of each litigant confronted each other in single combat, in the presence of the cross and using weapons which were marked with a cross. Others considered that the expression *exire ad crucem* alluded to the oath taken on the cross by each litigant. The hypothesis advanced by the learned Jérôme Bignon in 1665 seems the most plausible, that two notes were placed upon the altar, one of which was marked with a cross. A priest would then say a prayer and mix the notes. Whichever of the marriage partners drew the note bearing the cross was taken at his or her word.

The earliest reference to an examination of the genital parts occurs in the chapter 'Proposuisti de Probationibus', composed by Pope Gregory VIII at the end of the eleventh century in the form of an epistle to one of his bishops. The issue involved was that of proving the impotence of one particular man by establishing that his wife was still a virgin. The Pope approved the steps taken by his bishop and instructed him to place the matter in the hands of seven midwives.

A subsequent initiative taken by Innocent III (1198–1216) legitimised this type of medical examination. On this occasion, a woman had been accused of impotence by her husband. Wishing to be fully informed as to the situation, the bishop called upon several 'prudent and honest' matrons chosen from his diocese. He requested them to determine, with all due caution and on pain of endangering their immortal souls, whether the woman was capable of receiving the embraces of a husband. After a minute inspection, the midwives declared that she could never bear children because she had no genital organs.

Despite these developments, proof by *septima manus* did not fall into total abeyance. Pope Honorius III, the immediate successor to Innocent III, delivered a ruling in the case of a couple who, after eight years of marriage, of which three had effectively been passed in fraternal cohabitation, jointly declared that they had not succeeded in consummating the marriage. The Pope decided to corroborate their testimonial oath *per septimam manum* before granting them a separation.

However, the inadequacy of these traditional methods caused a progressive degradation of forensic procedures. Gradually, the doctrine of 'realism' triumphed. Proof of erection and trial by sexual congress came to be regarded by the ecclesiastical authorities as the supreme tests. At the same time the impotence trials, which had hitherto been marked by a certain restraint, degenerated, and, as a result of their improprieties, became the subject of sharp controversy.

It is practically impossible to establish the frequency with which these trials took place. The few dozen recorded cases give us perhaps only the pale reflection of a prodigious reality, but that is only a subjective interpretation. We must therefore rely upon the testimony of the commentators.

It would seem that from the sixteenth century onwards, the trickle of impotence trials took on the proportions of a tidal wave – an entirely new phenomenon. According to Tagereau, 'separations for impotency of men are today more frequent than they have ever been, though there are not today more impotents than in the past.' This was not a coincidence. Trial by congress, which had only recently been introduced into France, was so uncertain a procedure, and so unfavourable to husbands, that the conjugal bond or its rupture became dependent upon the goodwill of the wives: 'this path being easy and assured to follow their desires, due to the form of proceeding that is observed in the trials . . . As a result of which there are a quantity of such trials in the Church courts, the which were rare before the introduction of congress,' Tagereau explains.

The misogynistic overtones are more pronounced in the writings of Anne Robert:

The impudence of women is in our day so great that there is now nothing more common in trials and at the Court than the complaints of women and lascivious demands for the dissolution of their marriages.

For the lawyer Sébastien Roulliard, the general corruption of morals was responsible for the recent boom in impotence trials:

The corruptions of the times have given free rein to such procedures, whereas during the twelve hundred years past, when modesty would have possessed the souls and covered the visages of the matrons of France, hardly would there have been as many trials as in our day are frequent and daily occurrences.

Two centuries later, Maître Begon was to speak of 'ten thousand verdicts delivered during the seventeenth century.'

Finally, the frequency of impotence trials between the beginning of the sixteenth and the end of the eighteenth centuries was such as to leave an indelible memory during the early nineteenth century. 'It grieves us,' wrote the forensic doctor Fodéré, 'to note that of recent years the sessions of the parliamentary courts have been almost wholly given over to obscene lawsuits,' to the extent that, according to the testimony of the assistant public prosecutor Cochin, the inside of the courtrooms 'would soon contain a greater populace of discontented couples than the uncommon nature of any case had ever attracted of inquisitive citizens.'

It is probably necessary to qualify these statements, which are obviously tainted by prejudice. The exaggerations are patently obvious in the case of authors who, in the name of the cause they espouse, criticise this type of procedure and barely conceal their nostalgia for a time when such trials did not exist. In this spirit Doctor Fodéré tried to exalt the institution of divorce, which had succeeded in diverting couples from these odious litigious practices.

But the testimony of contemporaries is no less significant as evidence: undeniably, something had changed. Moreover, this change is easier to note than to explain. The 'will to knowledge', the impulse to probe the individual to the inmost recesses of his being, certainly operated as a stimulus. Here, Michel Foucault has very ably revealed the mechanisms which provoked the explosion of a discourse of sexuality during the sixteenth century. In this context, the dissemination of printed books – particularly confessors' manuals and theological treatises on impotence – is clearly relevant. Factums, which were printed in their thousands, made the trials a matter of common knowledge.

In addition, the new forensic procedures assured the trials a wide audience and prestige which they had previously lacked.

We must also allow a certain credibility to Tagereau's theory. Proof of erection and trial by congress were far too favourable to childless wives for a certain proportion of the latter not to have exploited in their own interests the weaknesses of a marriage system which was eminently misogynistic.

Whatever the reasons, impotence trials henceforth occupied the centre of the stage, and took place in an atmosphere of unhealthy curiosity and spectacular publicity, 'to the sound of public hue and cry', as one commentator put it. To use the expression of the chronicler Mathieu Marais, 'all and sundry run as if to a fire' to witness the proceedings. There was no comparable fascination with cases of bigamy or clandestine marriage. It was not merely the scabrous character of these proceedings which accounted for the public attention they received, for the theologians deliberately generated a public and even provocative atmosphere around the trials. Fevret offered an effortless justification of this. Since marriages are contracted amid great pomp and ceremony, it is therefore only reasonable that they should not be allowed to be dissolved in secret. Evidence flooded in from all quarters, and the trials soon began to take on the character of side-shows at a fairground.

A surgeon from La Rochelle, Jacques Mériaut, was accused of impotence by his wife. He volunteered for trial by congress. According to the account of his lawyer, Julien Peleus, 'this case, as being public and of great import, was conducted amidst much expectation and an astounding multitude of people.'

Marie de Corbie lodged a complaint against the impotence of Etienne de Bray by 'notices published in divers churches of the city of Paris, the which were full of calumnies and scandals.'

Towards the end of the seventeenth century, a young man from Issoudun requested a separation from his wife who had never been able to tolerate his attentions and who, at the very mention of the words 'husband' or 'marriage', would be seized with severe convulsions and spasms, 'her eyes rolling and turning upwards'. The ecclesiastical judge ordered a public examination of the unfortunate woman. 'The assembled company was numerous,' wrote the surgeon de Blegny, 'and composed of several persons of much standing, among whom was Madame the Intendant, who possessed all the delicacy of spirit of which her sex is capable.'

And in 1713, Maître Begon, the lawyer of Marie Magdeleine Mascranni, described 'the great troop of companions and courtiers that the Duc de Tresmes dragged along to the hearings' in which his son, the Marquis de Gesvres, was faced with the task of clearing himself of an accusation of impotence. Saint-Simon left an eloquent account of this trial:

It would be difficult to convey the scenes which did occur in the course of this affair. Well-known and even eminent personages turned up at the hearings to entertain themselves: places were reserved from early in the morning. People appeared, and came away with stories which then became the subject of every conversation. The poor Gesvres thought they would die from vexation and shame, and did thoroughly repent of having engaged in such a combat. It lasted a long time, constantly fuelled by new absurdities, and did end only with the life of the Marquise de Gesvres. It was commonly believed that the fault had not been entirely on her side, and her husband has somewhat confirmed this notion by not having contemplated remarriage these thirty years.

Impotence trials were in fashion, and to accommodate this the assistant public prosecutor requested – not without irony, and in the midst of a parliamentary session – that the city of Paris should 'enlarge the courts, extend their floor space, and dismantle the barriers intended to hold back the crowd . . .'

Under such circumstances, it is hardly surprising that the accused should have become a universal laughing stock and target for ridicule. 'Behold him exposed to the contumely and mockery of all and sundry,' wrote Julien Peleus. 'His fellow men hold him in abhorrence as an unfortunate encounter, and he cannot leave to posterity any image or remembrance of his person . . .'

But also, and perhaps to an even greater extent, it was by the austere pens of the magistrates that the seal of notoriety was stamped upon these sombre trials. The factums on the trials of Quellenec, De Bray, De Brosses, De Gesvres, Michel and Pochet proliferated and were swept by their thousands into the hands of an avid public. The De Gesvres trial alone produced at least twenty factums. Reports of medical examinations, which revelled in details, were also made public with complacency. Never did private parts have less privacy than those of the Marquis de Gesvres or Jacques François Michel. Even the outlying districts were given over to the curiosity of the public: François Michel's haemorrhoids provoked bizarre digressions in the speeches of the experts and lawyers.

In 1712, the subject of impotence trials forced itself upon the attention of that august institution, the Paris medical faculty, where Pierre Antoine Lepy defended the eloquently phrased thesis: *We ought never to despair of the capacity for love in a young man who is provided with all the necessary organs.* The choice of such a subject owed nothing to chance. On the contrary, it was a topic on everyone's lips, for the De Gesvres case was then in full swing. There was a packed audience to hear the debate, and the jury was hand-picked. Various eminent personalities of the day were present, including Michel Procope Couteau, Jean Claude Adrien Helvetius and François Vernage. As a final glorification of the occasion, the thesis was published in the form of an introduction to the famous *General Collection of Documents Relating to the Trial of the Marquis de Gesvres.*

What is more, the public took an active part in the trials. In the De Langey case, the women of Paris declared themselves in favour of the Marquis, at first, and then came out in favour of his wife. When Marie Magdeleine Mascranni brought a case against her husband, her lawyer noted:

Everyone threw themselves on the side of privilege and fortune. The intimates of Madame de Gesvres did in no wise consult their loyalty to her when they took sides. To support from afar a duke and peer of the realm was more attractive than to support and stand by a simple girl, though of distinguished family: thus did glamour prevail.

The tide of opinion turned, however, and by failing in all his attempts to prove his virility, the Marquis de Gesvres lost the support of his public.

The impotence trials extended beyond the courtrooms and invaded the streets, the salons, the court. They afforded an ideal subject for derision, and stimulated the invention of the wits about town. At the beginning of the seventeenth century, the medical examination of the genitals of the treasurer, Etienne de Bray, gave a particular stimulus to the mediocre

talents of several poets. A number of sonnets resulted, one of
which was published in 1947 in Brantôme's *Les Dames
Galantes*:
There was a most charming pleasantry made at the court, a noble lady
did read it aloud herself and gave it to me, when I did dine with her.
Some held that a lady had penned it, others a man. The sonnet goes
thus:

> *Among the Doctors of Paree, the most Renowned*
> *In Knowledge, Science, Practice and Doctrine*
> *– For judging all that fails in couples Androgyne –*
> *These by de Bray and his good wife were found.*
>
> *As for de Bray, he chose the three least dear:*
> *Le Court, Pietre, l'Endormy; his wife, refined,*
> *The four most expert in the art of Medicine*
> *(Le Grand, Le Gros, Duret and Vigoureux) did sign.*
>
> *By this we judge which of the twain will victor*
> *Be, and if Le Grand will thrash Le Court*
> *And if Le Gros, Duret, will lose to Pietre, or l'Endormy to*
> *Vigoureux.*
>
> *De Bray, that has but few upon his side,*
> *Deformities as gross as any husband can abide,*
> *Will be nonsuit – unless the good law do preside.*

The poem was found written in manuscript at the end of the
factum on De Bray's trial, in the Bibliothèque Nationale. Henri
Sauval emphasised the notoriety of the poem when he quoted it
in his *Chronique Scandaleuse de Paris* (1722): 'Among the
great quantity of verses that were composed to mock this
subject, it was considered to be an excellent example.'

The De Langey case unleashed a similar excess of satirical
spirit. 'Verses were composed about the affair,' wrote Tallemant des Réaux, 'that sinned against the truth, but expressed a
great quantity of filth.' On the morning after the trial, one
particular verse addressed to Louis XIV's minister Daillé was
on everyone's lips, sung to the tune of 'Maréchal Lampon':

Monsieur Daillé, please open up your door;
Grief overcomes me, I can take no more;
For I am Langey, who comes to find retreat;
For I am Langey, whom congress has defeated.

The De Langey trial also formed the subject of some of the poems collected by Gustave Brunet in his *Nouveau Siècle de Louis XIV ou Choix de chansons historiques et satiriques de 1634 à 1712* (1857). For example:

At last De Langey you must quit the Fray
For as a Soldier you are naught but Clay
Now all Men do see your Disarray
But None has witnessed your Triumphal Day.

Cease therefore to rail at Humankind,
Admit the fault lies in your own weak Spine;
Had you but mounted once unto the Breach
Such Labours might have won you many a Speech.

The Night was calm, the Port was clear to aim for,
You needed but some small degree of Vigour
With which you might have sailed into this Harbour
And thereby saved your Goods, your Monies and your Honour.

Yet it was probably the De Gesvres case that brought poetic inspiration to its fever pitch. The *Chansonnier* in the Bibliothèque Nationale offers a wide choice, of which the following are two examples:

Of a certain young Marquis it's said
He did nothing but sleep when in bed;
His wife stormed and cried:
'What a life do I lead,
What a villainous monster I've wed!'

So she ran to her parents at last
And raged and did take them to task:
'I'll never have children,
So now I must leave him,
And this my Confessor has passed.

'I insist that the magistrates listen,
For my marriage demands dissolution;
They must hear out my lawyers,
Ignore the World's rumours,
And heed my Confessor's permission.

'When you plough for a Husband, beware
Of those Marquis whose Members are tares;
I've paid a cruel price
I'm a Maid though a Wife
And these lines must suffice as my Heirs.'

In a Factum penned against a young Marquis
Begon, the sour and scathing Jurisconsult
Did sting, tear apart, vex and insult
A celebrated Writer praised by all Paris.

He reproached him and what's more did prove
Him to be a mediocre Physician
And an even worse Theologian.
The Public, disabused, did credit Begon and approve

His act: the worse is sooner believed than the better.
As for me, of this Begon I do frankly disapprove,
For though the Writer Arrault may be a Fool
The Jurisconsult ought to respect his Elder.

Under these circumstances, it is easy to imagine the fairground atmosphere that dominated the impotence trials.

The De Langey case, in particular, provoked a general atmosphere of hilarity and elation which was clearly directed at the expense of the unfortunate Marquis. A hubbub permeated the whole of Paris, and at times the collective mood took on the dimensions of a vast release of popular feeling, punctuated here and there by anti-aristocratic overtones. A few years later, the De Gesvres trial provoked the same reactions. On the other hand, the cases involving Jean François Michel and Lahure-Pochet, despite their fame, left plebeian sensibilities untouched.

For over two years, from 1657 to 1659, Parisians vicariously lived out the dramas which afflicted the Marquis de Langey and his wife, Marie de Saint-Simon. Crowds gathered spontaneously, witticisms flew back and forth, songs were sung, verses recited, caricatures scribbled. Tallemant des Réaux left a sparkling account of this epic and unforgettable jubilee. It would doubtless be rash to take Tallemant's venomous account literally, but there is nevertheless something authentic about the atmosphere of turmoil and excitement which pervades his 'anecdotal history of Madame de Langey'.

When the affair broke out, De Langey was looked on as a persecuted hero. A very handsome man, he was at first idolised by the Parisians. 'Alas, whom may we trust in future?' exclaimed Madame de Franquetot-Caraba upon seeing him. The 'haranguers and other women' waited for him at the exit of Châtelet, where his interrogation was taking place. (Since De Langey was a Protestant, the trial was heard by the High Court of Paris, not the ecclesiastical court.) 'May it please God for me to have a husband who looks like that,' the women were heard to mutter. The experts responsible for examining the genitals of Marie de Saint-Simon could find no apparent sign of an intact virginity. Upon reading the report, Renevilliers-Galand, the advisor to the Châtelet, could not help crying out in admiration: 'It cannot be denied that Langey has done a fair amount of work with his ten fingers these past four years.'

Here the accuser was in the dock, and, while the women 'did heap all manner of abuse upon her', her husband was loudly triumphing. 'From this time up until the trial by congress, all the women were for De Langey; besides, he said nothing against his wife. He was to be seen in public much more than hitherto, and it was said that this affair had given him new spirit.'

With the expectation of a favourable verdict, the Marquis ought perhaps to have remained content with the flattering outcome of the examination. However, carried away by his popularity and goaded by the wish to restore his battered ego, he rashly requested a trial by congress.

Instantly, the whole of Paris exploded with excitement. 'Everywhere people spoke only of that ... the vaudevilles could sing of nothing else.' But scepticism carried the day in the end. De Langey found himself lumbered with the nickname 'marquis du congrès', and doubts began to circulate as to his capacity to withstand the inhibitive ordeal of trial by congress. The controversy in any case rapidly developed, and the betting was brisk. The minister Gache and the doctor L'Aimonon supported De Langey, on admittedly fragile premises: 'The former did trust that De Langey was too God-fearing to lie in such a matter, and the latter held that he was of too good a family on both sides to lie. Meniot, the doctor, said jestingly that the others were De Langey's two c... [testicles]: M. L'Aimonon the right one, and M. Gache the left one.' A similar sentiment was expressed by Madame de Sévigné: 'As for you,' she observed drily to De Langey, 'your trial is in your breeches.' When the civil lieutenant, Le Camus, took De Langey's side, it was apparently only to please Madame de Lavardin. And Madame d'Olonne was pleased to overbid wildly in her support of the Marquis: 'I would so like to be condemned to trial by congress,' she sighed gallantly.

The fateful day arrived. The trial was to take place at the house of a certain bath-house owner named Turpin. 'Madame de Lavardin and Madame de Sévigné, friends of the civil lieutenant, were esconced in a coach two doors away, where he was to find them afterwards; their laughter could be heard from the end of the street.' As for the intrepid candidate himself, 'he arrived proclaiming his victory, for all the world as if he were already *in*: never has there been such boasting.'

But in the end – failure! And the piteous circumstances in which the unfortunate Marquis succumbed were obligingly divulged and widely publicised. 'The morning after, De Langey was the sole topic of conversation. Never were so many obscenities uttered on a Shrove Tuesday. The minister Gache was so confused that you would have said it was he to whom this misfortune had arrived.' The occasion was a feast for the women. Those 'that had been for De Langey were confounded – he is a vile creature, they said, let us speak no more of him.'

The Marquis made one request after another for a retrial, to no avail. He lost the case. 'After which, he had the effrontery to attend a ball; upon his being asked to dance, out of malice, there was a singular outburst of hootings.' Thereafter, 'Langey' became synonymous with 'impotent', to the extent that, when his grandmother Téligny died, he changed his name to the Marquis de Téligny. 'But he remained a Langey for all that,' observed Tallemant cynically.

However, his hour of revenge was yet to come. Breaking the interdictions which had been placed upon him, he remarried a few years later, a certain Mademoiselle de Navailles. Venomous as ever, Tallement noted 'that this time 'tis a strange bird he has chosen . . . thin, old and dark.' But this did not prevent De Langey providing his new wife with seven children, one after another!

'There you are,' he exclaimed to Benserade, who had often mocked him, 'despite your tasteless jests, my wife gave birth to a sturdy son only yesterday.'

'But, sir,' replied Benserade, 'nobody has ever had any doubts about your wife.'

However, the De Langey affair was only the beginning.

We have already seen that, behind the burlesque façade, all the elements of individual tragedy were present in the impotence trials. But not all the trials provoked the same farcical frenzy. The Quellenec case, by contrast, took place in an atmosphere whose sobriety was such as to confer upon it the intensity of a

Greek tragedy. However, the impotence of Charles de Quellenec did not thereby lose any of the public character generic to these trials. In this case it was the grandees of the kingdom of France and Navarre who, far from the noise and sensationalism of the marketplace, chose to embroil themselves in the affair, and managed in the end to confer upon it an unprecedented notoriety.

On 20 June 1568, outside La Rochelle, a Breton nobleman, Baron Charles de Quellenec, married a girl of twelve years of age, Catherine de Parthenay de Soubise. Their conjugal happiness was to last only two years. Imperceptibly, a rumour of the Baron's impotence began to spread. It seems that the girl's mother was the first to make the affair public in the higher echelons of the aristocracy. She personally informed the Queen of Navarre, Jeanne d'Albret, of her son-in-law's incapacity. On two separate occasions, she attempted without success to intervene with a view to securing an annulment of the marriage. At this point, Madame de Soubise turned for help to Henri de Navarre, the future Henri IV.

Irritated and anxious to let matters die down, Charles de Quellenec meanwhile retired to Brittany. His wife followed him, perhaps under constraint. At this point Admiral Coligny interfered in the business, requesting the Baron to return Catherine to her mother.

Henceforth, the affair was to enjoy considerable publicity in the French court. A series of letters arrived from the young wife, each contradicting the other. Some of them, perhaps written under pressure from her husband, conveyed his opposition to an annulment. Elsewhere, mother and daughter managed to express their real thoughts by writing in between the lines in Greek or Latin, using lemon or orange juice which was invisible until the paper was held in front of a flame.

At the beginning of 1571, Madame de Soubise decided to go to the court. Immediately, Charles de Quellenec wrote to de

Niort, the minister of La Rochelle, requesting him to use his authority to dissuade her. The mother-in-law, in her desire to snatch Catherine from captivity, now turned to the Queen Mother, Catherine de Médicis. Moreover, she obtained from the ministers of the Protestant Church a written consultation which she sent to her son-in-law, in which the marriage of her daughter was denounced in the most violent terms as an 'infamous union', a 'blemish' and a 'sacrilege'.

At the same time, the Queen of Navarre and Admiral Coligny were attempting to have a private interview with Catherine de Parthenay. Coligny's personal messenger read out the admiral's letter to Quellenec, in which he declared himself convinced of the good faith of Madame de Soubise and maintained that the steps she was taking were justified.

The affair had got out of control. The Baron gave up his defensive strategy. He decided to confront his mother-in-law openly, at the French court. He sent his wife to La Rochelle, where the admiral advised her, without success, to request an annulment. Prompted by the failure of her husband, Madame de Coligny took the matter in hand. She informed the King of Navarre of what had taken place, and asked him to take Catherine under his protection.

Now events took a tragic turn. Madame de Soubise managed to have her daughter locked up, while Quellenec, taking up the challenge, decided on a frontal counter-attack. He served a writ on his mother-in-law and demanded reparation for the calumnies that she had heaped upon him. On Tuesday 11 September 1571, the case was heard in camera. Unfortunately, nobody will ever know what happened, for the account is incomplete and breaks off just at this point.

However, the anonymous author did leave some points of reference which make it possible for us to trace the sequel:

'Catherine de Soubise uncovered herself,' which evidently refers to a medical examination.

'It is our intention to test the capacities of the lord du Pont by physicians and surgeons. Request is made to have him lie with the girl.' The allusion to trial by congress here is quite plain. Two explanations are nevertheless possible. Either the medical examination of Catherine was inconclusive and necessitated a trial by congress, or the young woman was deemed to be a virgin and her husband volunteered for congress in order to exonerate himself.

The trial took place at Blois. Gaspard de Coligny arrived on time, which indicates that peers of the realm were on occasion capable of showing themselves attentive to small matters. The case, however, took a turn for the worse when the Baron claimed that he was the victim of a spell. Catherine was locked up in the house of the 'Dame de Bouillon'. Then, suddenly, the affair came to a bloody end, when Charles de Quellenec died as a victim of the massacre of Saint Bartholomew, on the night of 23 August 1572.

Yet there was a lamentable epiloque, and the case was finally closed amidst gales of laughter. According to Bayle's *Dictionnaire*, the Queen Catherine de Médicis, in a fit of unhealthy curiosity, 'gave orders to search out the body of Soubise, a gentleman suspected of impotence, and, after it had been found, she did examine the genital parts thereof with great cries of mirth, in the presence of a large company of her ladies-in-waiting.'

It was precisely this kind of indecent publicity surrounding the impotence trials which prompted several commentators to denounce their obscene nature. Certainly the proceedings were inherently provocative. As Sébastien Roulliard noted: 'If divine law does prohibit a wife from fondling or precipitating herself upon her husband's genitals, with even less reason should it countenance the respondent divulging that she has some resentment against those of her spouse.' That such an accusation should come from a girl who claimed to be a virgin was regarded as the height of indecency. In this connection, a text by John of Salisbury was often cited, which concerned a lawyer who had placed one plaintiff wife in an awkward situation:

He did demand of her, in the presence of several witnesses, whether her husband had caressed or kissed or embraced her. She replied that he had. 'And who then did tell you that this does not suffice?' he asked her. 'Where did you learn the rest? If your virginity be intact, as you do proclaim, you ought not to have any awareness that your husband is impotent; and if you do know him to be impotent, this is a sign that you have essayed what other men have to offer.' He did press her in this manner as to make her blush and admit that she could make no satisfactory answer to such embarrassing questions.

Wives who embarked upon the adventure of an impotence trial automatically compromised themselves. Most often they were accused of succumbing to physical desire. According to Bayle's *Dictionnaire*, it was damnation enough for a woman

to confess publicly that she cannot contain herself. For every woman who institutes such proceedings [against her husband] does declare to all and sundry that she has such a defect: her action remains on record and she does become an object of derision to wags and farcers and even an object of dread to her future husband. For if he does find himself compelled to make long voyages abroad, or if he suffers a protracted illness, upon what basis will he trust the virtue of a wife that has admitted her incontinence in broad daylight and before the whole world?

Hence these unfortunate women became, in the words of Dr Pierre Sue, 'the laughing stock of one and all'. This was all the more true since the trials to which they submitted themselves were a deliberate outrage to public decorum: 'These procedures are so contrary to modesty, to that virtue which is the crown and ornament of the fair sex, that we cannot esteem any woman that is capable of undergoing them.'

Even the questioning of the couple was regarded as an

indecency, because 'it is perforce inevitable that the ears of the judges be assailed by all manner of obscenities.'

In more general terms, it was the unhealthy atmosphere pervading the ecclesiastical courts which Boursault denounced in his *Lettres Nouvelles*. He addressed the Bishop de Langres as follows:

On more than one occasion have I been struck by the fact that you Monsignori and prelates do suffer priests to be the magistrates of the ecclesiastical courts, or that you do not insist such proceedings be heard in private, on account of the frankness which is to be heard therein and which does in nearly all cases degenerate into obscenity. For myself I have never been so curious as to be present at one of these occasions, but I have heard them spoken of by divers persons, and what they have related to me has invariably seemed so loose as to make it appear that these are proceedings from which all modesty has been discarded. I do need no other evidence for this than the matter which is contained in these verses:

> In one Officiality
> Some days ago, a maid
> Of passing beauty and well-made,
> Robust and hale as horse,
> Discarding all propriety
> Did claim an aged doctor had taken her by force
> And that he needs must hang – or be her spouse.
> 'But how,' replied the judge, 'could he have ta'en you thus?
> For you are strong, yourself should have defended
> To scratch, disfigure and him o'erwhelm.'
> 'I have, Sir, for my part,'
> Said she, 'some force when I do quarrel
> But none when I do laugh.'

Maître Vertamont was inspired by the same sentiments as Boursault, when he acted as counsel for Magdeleine Pigousse in the appeal case brought before the High Court of Paris by Nicolas Jaillot in 1666. According to him,

There is nothing more opposed to the sanctity of the Sacerdocy than these filthy and shameful interrogations to which the most private matters that exist between husband and wife are subjected. For it is in no wise sufficient that a priest have a pure heart, he must also have chaste ears: how then may he legitimately listen to matters concerning which he is obliged by the nature of his office to be ignorant?

Tribute must be paid to the lucidity of Boursault and Vertamont. By condemning the shameless practices of the ecclesiastical courts, they were the only commentators implicitly to exonerate the women compromised by such cases. Their denunciations of the obscene character of the impotence trial provoked an extraordinary profusion of aggressive pleas on its behalf. However, by an astonishing shift of responsibility, the women who complained of their husbands were seen as the ones at fault, rather than the Church magistrates who wallowed in the mire of public scandal. Clearly, for a wife to have recourse to canonical structures which had been laboriously formulated by theologians was neither a crime nor a sin. But it was perhaps more in her interest to remain unaware of their existence. Thus according to the annotator of Bayle's *Dictionnaire*, although there existed certain 'actions' which in themselves were neither sinful nor branded as infamous

de facto or *de jure*; nonetheless, because it were better far to refrain from them than to proceed with them, they do carry a certain aura which suffices to tarnish a reputation.

This was a cruel dilemma. Morally speaking, the wife of an impotent man found herself in a debilitating impasse, where she was deemed culpable whether she took action or whether she refrained from taking action. If she suffered in silence, she was regarded as a prey to sinfulness and the lascivious furies of a counterfeit husband. If she made a show of her torment, she became the focus of public outrage. Whatever she did, the inexorable misogynistic stranglehold tightened its grip upon her.

Was the fate of such a woman less enviable than that of her

impotent partner? This is entirely debatable. For it was only rarely that a husband triumphed over the proof of erection and the trial by congress. Thus magistrates championed impotent husbands with a cynical zeal, without having to forfeit any of the misogynistic ardour which motivated them.

Some authors, it is true, undertook the defence of impotence trials and of the women who resorted to them. In a work dedicated to the rehabilitation of congress, the magistrate Bouhier rose up in indignation against the prejudices which discriminated against a plaintiff wife.

Was she not otherwise abandoned to the impure flames of a passion which could not satisfy itself? 'If she does suffer willingly the odious tauntings of her counterfeit husband, she is accused of a crime. If she resists him, she does expose herself to his fits of anger and his rage . . . Is it not in all cases praise-worthy for her to flee the perils of incontinence to which she is exposed by the actions of a licentious husband? . . .' She is deprived of all hope of maternity, and she is in danger of losing her immortal salvation.

Maître Begon developed these arguments in a series of pleas which he wrote in defence of Marie Magdeleine Mascranni. When the De Gesvres affair broke out . . .

. . . the dull-witted holier-than-thous were scandalised, the vain-headed prudes were shocked, and the light-headed and thoughtless windbags (a race which constitutes the larger part of human-kind) argued the matter endlessly back and forth.

From all sides Magdeleine Mascranni was accused of suffering from a bilious nature. She was not, however, unaware of the problems of an impotence trial when she embarked upon this course of action,

but when the fire has spread to all parts of the house, and when the only remaining path for saving your skin is through a door that may be reached only by penetrating the thick of the smoke and the heaps of debris and rubbish, do you then have qualms about dirtying your feet or stinking out your clothes?

In spite of such arguments, women who offered themselves up to these ordeals were only ever partially rehabilitated. By taking the edge off the more deplorable side-effects of the impotence trial, it would seem that many jurists and theologians were primarily concerned with ensuring the survival of an institution which permitted them to appease their secret fascination while at the same time consolidating their secular power and rights of intervention in the intimacies of married life. In fact, the martyrdom of a frustrated wife was of little concern to them, and the protection which they afforded wives accused of shamelessness had no basis in a feminist ethos.

The misogynistic tendencies which covertly entrenched themselves during the eighteenth century, in a more or less subtle and discreet but obsessive and incisive manner, had erupted a century earlier in an amorphous mass of vulgar formulations about the nature of women. They were characterised as impatient, cunning, false, lascivious, inconstant, and so on. In view of which it was advocated that impotence cases should be instigated only by the marital authority – the husband. 'The man is ruler of the woman,' wrote Sébastien Roulliard, 'and should get the better of her by employing this prerogative.' The jurist Anne Robert considered it salutary to reflect upon the example of the ancient Romans. For centuries, only husbands had been entitled to draw up a divorce agreement, because 'the ancients were very cognisant of the effrontery and impudence of women, and did accordingly essay to hold in check and as it were bridle this untameable creature, owing to the flightiness and audacity of her sex . . . For if she be given her head, she is apt to be cruel, ambitious, and desirous of grandeur.' This is why the institution of divorce was thought to have degenerated when women were accorded the same rights as men. As Seneca remarked, 'dissoluteness, insolence and abuse all proceed from that cause.'

Besides, was it possible to place one's trust in 'so fickle and so fragile a sex'? Sébastien Roulliard noted that

by a special law of Moses it was forbidden to accept the testimony of a woman against her own husband, not only as a thing which tended to corrupt standards of behaviour and transgress the limits of modesty, but also because women do lack a strong and solid enough judgement to support such a testimony; for although 'tis an argument arising from an ill-provided marriage bed, they do attempt to supplement it by an excess of rancour and hatred.

Their impatience was in itself suspect, in that they relinquished separation procedures for ill-treatment, 'this being a long, difficult and hazardous process.' Impotence trials provided them with a far more expedient and effective way out of marriage, according to Tagereau. Equally, women were regarded as responsible for the continued success of these shameful customs. 'Their restless appetites do provoke husbands into trial by congress and the amatory combats of Venus,' wrote Anne Robert. An addiction to change was often considered to be their only motivation. In 1577, a man by the name of Mériaut was charged with being impotent. He subsequently vanished without trace for nine years. Upon his return he learnt that his marriage had been dissolved and that his wife had remarried. 'Oh how foolish men are,' lamented his lawyer, 'to leave their wives at home when undertaking a long voyage! Incontinent as women are by nature, they do consign their husbands to oblivion and their affections do cool as rapidly as that side of the bed in which their husbands had slept.'

This unfortunate female penchant for novelty inspired the surgeon Guillemeau to write an even more caustic tract:

There are but too many women of a more than brutish nature, so much so that, were we to allow ourselves to be deceived by them, they would be happy to change husbands every month . . . Women are all too shameless and haughty by nature, all too covetous of novelties, all too changeable and unresolved . . .

In view of which, Guillemeau advised women to follow the example of horses:

The insolence and lasciviousness of womankind must needs be bridled. Horses, on the contrary, do love the partners with whom they do happen to be harnessed under the same yoke, in such manner that if one is changed, the other does refuse any longer to pull.

Unquestionably, the impotence trial developed under conditions which encouraged the expression of misogynistic sentiments. Embroiled in this poisonous system, women were remorselessly crushed by a legal machinery which was at the same time biased in their favour. This was only an apparent contradiction: hatred for impotent men prevailed over that for the female sex. Nevertheless, implicated at all levels, the wife could be separated from her husband only at the cost of a cruel victimisation. The frequency of the trials as well as their shameless and sensational character were attributed to women. As we have seen, women were held responsible for the introduction of improper forensic procedures, and, as we shall see later on, the repeated interference by mothers-in-law, though it was in many cases motivated by the worst intentions, was depicted in an unnecessarily and profoundly misogynistic light.

Indeed, by mercilessly underlining the marginal status of the impotent, this type of trial served to establish 'structures of exclusion' which operated for women as effectively as for their deficient husbands.

5

Legal procedures

It is difficult to understand how, throughout the entire *Ancien Régime*, the dissolution of the sacrament of marriage could have been a matter for the independent jurisdiction of the Church. At the same time, this apparently exclusive prerogative sparked off a controversy, albeit a hidden controversy: ecclesiastical and secular authorities confronted each other without ever coming openly to blows. Resuming the arguments put forward by Vincent Hotman at the beginning of the seventeenth century, Michel Roussel in 1625 maintained that impotence trials ought not to be the sole responsibility of the ecclesiastical courts.

This line of thinking was illustrated, as late as the eighteenth century, by Pierre Le Ridant. According to this jurist, the competency of Church magistrates in judging impotence trials was a recent phenomenon which was not supported by any tradition. Over the centuries, he argued, the Church had exercised no jurisdiction whatsoever in this domain.

The prerogatives of secular law, on the other hand, were based upon a different set of criteria. For although the marriage of an impotent was a profanation of the holy sacrament, the Church could not proclaim the nullity of such a union without assuming the right to give rulings on the status of citizens within the civil and political order. And this right came within the exclusive jurisdiction of civil law.

The importance of this 'civilist' tendency is borne out by the *Grande Encyclopédie* of 1777, which discreetly but effectively denounced the Church's usurpation of these prerogatives.

In fact, the question of competency came within the

framework of a larger debate. From the fifteenth century onwards, the State had been endeavouring to break down the Church's sovereignty in marital affairs and to hold in check its exclusive prerogative on matters of matrimonial legislation. Within a very short time an understanding was reached. From the sixteenth century, kings took it upon themselves to give rulings on marriages, by means of a series of edicts and ordinances.

As early as the fourteenth century, legists had made inroads upon the ecclesiastical monopoly by extending their jurisdiction to cover a number of circumstances pertaining to marriage (such as financial settlements in cases of annulment, rulings on the legitimacy of children and on cases of adultery).

The introduction of appeals against corrupt or abusive practices during the sixteenth century would appear to have satisfied the supporters of both sides. An area of competency was formally ceded to the ecclesiastical courts, but henceforth the recourse to this appeal was still possible in cases where the laws, the customs of the land or the canons of the Church were seen to be transgressed. When this happened, the matter would be referred to the High Courts and the corrupt practice was liable to be annulled.

In other words, this one-sided and paternalistic agreement ensured the subordination of ecclesiastical justice to secular justice. The frequency of these appeals and the proliferation of categories of abuse confirmed the ascendancy of the High Courts. A rejected appeal or a case which was referred to the ecclesiastical court did not necessarily reinforce the power of the Church judge. One suspects that the High Courts reserved the important cases for themselves and handed the minor cases over to the ecclesiastical courts.

This explains why the conflict outlined in the eighteenth century by Le Ridant could never have turned into a protracted public confrontation, and why impotence trials – with the exception of the most important ones – were to remain within the Church's jurisdiction.

As for the trial itself, it evolved within a formalistic and hieratic framework. In its earlier forms, it was of the utmost simplicity. A petition was lodged, after which a summons was issued requesting the parties concerned to appear before the ecclesiastical court in order to undergo the traditional cross-examination. But the final verdict remained subject to the mandatory report drawn up by the physicians and surgeons after the forensic examination of the genitals.

Nevertheless, there was no standard or typical procedure. Moreover, certain individual case histories must be taken into account because of their incidental variations which became assimilated to the ideal schema: cases where the accused took to flight, where husband and wife both accused each other of impotence, where the findings of the experts were challenged, where two, three or even four medical examinations were required, where the reports of the experts were contradictory, or where a surgical operation changed the course of a particular case.

Thus impotence trials could vary in length, although on the whole they tended to be short. A trial which followed the ideal format would be settled in under three months. One well-documented case took seven and a half months. However, during this period the respondent absconded twice, and on both occasions it was necessary to call upon the services of the secular authorities to find him. Another case encountered numerous obstacles, in spite of which it was settled in under eight months. Although a further recorded case provides an example of a trial lasting three years, both parties had to undergo surgical operations during the course of it.

The brevity which characterised the trials was in fact spurious, and their apparent efficiency a mere illusion. For the courts wasted their energies upon formalities and minutiae.

The vain and obsessive use of the royal 'we', the endless recourse to obscure jargon, the display of glittering titles which recurs with monotonous regularity in all the court minutes – such devices served to augment the proceedings. The names of the ecclesiastical judge, the legal counsellors and the physicians and surgeons were constantly embellished with a pompous titular apparatus. The court accounts are littered with ponderous references to innumerable theological doctors, each cited by name, and an understanding of the accounts is further obstructed by their finicky preoccupation with detail. The most trivial matters are reported with meticulous care, and the reports of court hearings and medical examinations are studded with incongruous and irrelevant remarks. Thus, from this often incoherent verbiage the few elements which formed the actual substance of the trials can be extracted only with the greatest difficulty. The rest served to advance the personal ends of the Church judges.

All this redundant phrasemongering in fact constituted one of the foundations of their power within society. By grandiloquent prognostication and pompous formulae, by parading his titles and the support of the august doctors of theology who sat at his side, the ecclesiastical judge imposed his authority. He spent more time in justifying himself before the public and the court than he did in fulfilling his role as a judge. If one considers closely the basic procedural elements which are scattered here and there throughout the court minutes, it becomes clear that a case usually required no more than fifteen days to settle.

Three types of verdict could be reached at the end of an impotence trial:

1. The reports of the medical examinations could be favourable to the spouse accused of impotence, in which case the couple were 'condemned to live as man and wife'.

2. The accused could be deemed impotent as charged, in which case the judge annulled the marriage and 'prohibited the

couple from seeking out or consorting with each other'. The injured party was given permission to 'provide for him or herself elsewhere', while the impotent party was ordered to pay damages and contribute a sum in aid of the poor of the parish. Although he or she was also forbidden to remarry, this interdiction was so universally contravened that it would be pointless to list the 'impotent' individuals who entered into wedlock a second time.

3. Finally, the judge could order the couple to undertake the *triennium*, or three-year period of enforced cohabitation. Instituted by Justinian, this probationary test had been adopted by canon law and confirmed by Pope Celestine III (in the chapter 'Laudabilem extra de Frigidis'). However, the legitimacy of the *triennium* was not unanimously accepted by jurists. Some regarded it as a profanation of the holy sacrament, in the same way as the marriage of an impotent. Like fraternal cohabitation, did it not expose a defenceless wife to the rages of her humiliated husband, to the immodest excesses of an impotent man, or even to interference and corruption by a stranger who might be introduced as a proxy by her desperate husband? Thus in such cases enormous care was taken to 'sequestrate' the wife in the house of a friend or relative where, in the words of Boucher d'Argis, 'the husband is to be accorded the liberty of seeing and lying with her when it does please him.'

In fact, the *triennium* was only prescribed in very rare cases. According to the collections of court records, it was ordered only twice during the entire seventeenth century.

The procedure for lodging a petition was basically quite simple. Whatever confessions the protagonists volunteered of their own accord, it was nevertheless determined at a high level of moral and spiritual patronage that the reception facilities should operate in favour of the partner injured by the impotence of his or her spouse. The annulment of the sacrament thus depended, as did the prohibition to celebrate a marriage, exclusively upon the initiative of the partners themselves.

The unsatisfied wife would generally appear before the ecclesiastical judge confidently protected by the veil of her modesty and inspired by the worthiest sentiments. These were very familiar: a burning desire for motherhood, the torments of the flesh, the brutal and unbridled behaviour of a sexually deficient husband, the anguish and obsessive fear of being in a state of sin, and so on. Often in the course of the cross-examination, or in a tearful petition addressed to the court judge, the supplicant would recite a dramatic tale concerning the discovery of the incapacity which afflicted her partner:

Henriette from the town of L . . . does humbly beg and implore your worship, stating that on the third day of August 1683 she was married to Henry de Hou in the church of . . . , and having been in his company some fifteen days thereafter, she did remark that he had some defect in his person, since, far from showing himself as ready to consummate the aforesaid marriage, he did repeatedly avoid the supplicant, now on the pretext of divers indispositions, now pleading fatigue and now sleepiness, so as to make pass the occasion; but upon closer examination of his excuses, the aforesaid supplicant judged that they did doubtless proceed from strange causes . . .

Leaving aside the motives expressed so eloquently, we should examine more closely the hidden motivations of the plaintiffs. The pious façade often concealed sordid interests, or a straightforward desire for a change of partner. In some cases, partners divided by an irrevocable incompatibility of temperament colluded in order to break the bond which united them against their will.

In the majority of cases, it is true, a providential father confessor can be glimpsed over the shoulder of the plaintiff. For how else could the young woman presumed to be an innocent virgin explain the knowledge which made it possible for her to accuse her husband of impotence?

The confessor of Marie Magdeleine Mascranni seems to

have played a decisive role in the case brought against the
Marquis de Gesvres. Maître Begon wrote:

The father confessor of a newly married maid seldom omits to probe
the secrets of the marriage bed. Nor did the confessor of Madame de
Gesvres forget himself in this respect, and it was through the ignorance displayed by Madame de Gesvres, and through the host of
naiveties which did issue from her mouth, that her confessor did
discover the impotence of M. de Gesvres.

This confessor quickly brought to bear pressures which gave
him a discretionary power of intrusion upon the De Gesvres
marriage – a union which according to him was tainted with a
thousand impurities:

Which is why from the outset of the marriage he did refuse absolution
to Madame de Gesvres, the which did greatly astound her, for she was
unaware of the reasons for this refusal. But when the Theory of
marriage in all its entirety had substituted for the Mystery in her
dealings with her confessor, this was because this confessor did speak
too openly of such matters.

This interference was unauthorised, it is true; for, as we have
noted, the lodging of a petition for the annulment of a marriage
could originate only in the independent wish of the injured
party. But the law and logic of this were subject to infringe-
ments, and the direct or indirect interference by third parties
was not uncommon. The impotence of a brother or uncle was
sometimes cited by direct heirs or collaterals who felt they had
been wrongly cheated of their inheritance. By obtaining an
invalidation of the marriage, they naturally hoped to recover
their fortune. But according to jurists and theologians, such
lawsuits had little chance of being heard, and the rulings in
several specific cases furnish proof that this was so.

In 1577, Maître François d'Assis, a seventy-seven-year-old
Toulouse notary, married a seventeen-year-old chambermaid
by the name of Jacquette. In 1581, his young wife became a
mother. Soon afterwards, Maître d'Assis died, whereupon his

family immediately lodged a suit, claiming that the child was begotten not by the deceased but by a physician named Sallette with whom Jacquette had been living 'lecherously'. Moreover, her husband had by no means been ignorant of this liaison, for he had nicknamed his wife 'Sallette's whore'. The unfortunate d'Assis, ill and afflicted by 'the sweating sickness', had been unable to procreate. He 'was so stiff in his limbs that his chin did touch his knees and his backside did touch his heels.' The Toulouse High Court nevertheless decided in favour of Jacquette, ruling that 'relatives are not competent to contest the status of the child *et frigiditatem et impotentiam arguere* [and dispute questions of frigidity and impotence].'

In 1675, Marguerite Miron had a writ issued against her husband, Louis Breuillard, Count de Coursan, to appear before the ecclesiastical court of Sens on a charge of impotence. However, the Count was the father of three children baptised in his name. In spite of this the deposition was accepted. At this juncture, Marguerite Miron died. Her sister, the lady Jacquinot, lodged a petition requesting a certificate of repossession in her favour, together with permission to summons the Count. Once again, the deposition was accepted. The situation now involved a widower being prosecuted for impotence by his sister-in-law. A few days later, the unfortunate Count followed his wife to the grave, whereupon his son took up the proceedings in his father's name. The case was heard on appeal before the Paris High Court on 31 March 1678. The judges ruled that a charge of impotence was 'in no wise subject to being taken up by another party'. The proceedings initiated by the ecclesiastical judge were declared 'null and abusive', and the request of the lady Jacquinot was deemed 'inadmissible'.

On the other hand, proceedings initiated by a third party stood every chance of being crowned with success when they involved the question of standards of behaviour. The Marquis de Vaudy and his wife, Mademoiselle de Cheppy, had been granted an annulment by the ecclesiastical court of Saint-Germain. The collusion of the parties was nevertheless obvious. The wife's brother brought the case before the High Court of Paris, added to which the assistant public prosecutor Bignon also requested to be received as a third party 'appealing against a corrupt practice'. The petition of both third parties was heard, the annulment invalidated and the verdict of the ecclesiastical court declared to be null.

Another example is that of Pernette Marion, who, after eight years of married life, claimed that her husband, Antoine Gay, was impotent. The latter calmly confirmed his wife's statements, and the marriage was dissolved without any other form of trial. But Pernette proceeded to remarry, whereupon the family of her new husband successfully contested the marriage.

The risk of collusion was thus all too real, and it was not without reason that the surgeon Guillemeau and the jurist Boucher d'Argis denounced the dangers.

Finally, was a husband entitled to admit to impotence and bring a lawsuit against himself? Pothier posed this problem in its extreme form:

Maevius was a rich but ugly man. He married a young widow who was poor but beautiful, and provided her with a life allowance of one hundred livres. After three years of marriage, he declared himself to be congenitally impotent and requested the dissolution of the marriage. His wife maintained the contrary and requested that the marriage be confirmed. According to Pothier, both partners were helped and hindered by suppositions which cancelled each other out. In the husband's favour was the notion that to declare onself impotent was a shameful act, and rarely admitted without an inner struggle. In the wife's favour, it was difficult to believe that a pretty woman would wish to remain with an impotent man. On the other hand, it could be argued that Maevius, though physically capable of satisfying his sexual needs, had given up all hope of becoming a father and was now looking for a pretext to deprive his wife of her life allowance. Similarly, it could be argued against his wife that she might prefer the comforts of life to the joys of the conjugal act.

Thus, depending upon the merits of each case, the courts were alert to abuses and could often sense when the impotence trial was being exploited for personal ends. There were, after all, cases of women marrying impotent men solely in order to obtain damages later. Frequently diverted from its ostensible aims, the impotence trial became a façade for the most sordid transactions, and an ideal melting pot in which to concoct every variation on the basic theme of a spouse in search of freedom or collaterals excluded from their inheritance. Finally, in addition to serving as a pretext for the most disreputable of motivations, the trial was a platform for the darkest machinations of mothers-in-law.

Interventions by confessors, heirs or outsiders all seem relatively innocuous when compared to the part played by the mother-in-law in several trials. It was during the seventeenth century that this figure came to dominate the scene with increasing ferocity. Tagereau noted that in impotence cases 'the wives are aided and in most cases abetted by mothers discontented with their sons-in-law.' This view was shared by Julien Peleus, who held the Baron d'Argenton's mother-in-law largely responsible for the suit which Magdeleine de la Chastre brought against him, 'his wife having passed four years in his house with all docility and modesty, but rendered incontinent by the influence of her mother, did cast off this frame of mind, and abandon conjugal harmony for a state of the deepest enmity, as if she had drunk of the poisonous well of marital hatred.'

In the same spirit, one of Sébastien Rouillard's speeches for the defence of a husband accused of impotence turned into a blazing indictment of the latter's mother-in-law. In this case, he exclaimed, the mother-in-law had interposed herself 'to serve as the fuse to this gun, the fan to this furnace, the lance to this ulcer.' As for the daughter, 'had it not been for the importunate terrorising and outcries of her mother, she would never have allowed such a scandal to be made public.'

In another case, the lawyer of Etienne de Bray set out the facts in a manner which openly blamed Marie d'Alvergne, the mother-in-law of his client. Was it not she who, over-ambitious to have one of the King's counsellors and inspector of finances for a son-in-law, had pushed her daughter, Marie de Corbie, into marriage? From the start of his engagement, however, De Bray had sensed that his marriage would soon be steeped in an unwholesome atmosphere. Had not Marie d'Alvergne had her own first husband poisoned by his son, who was still languishing in the galleys serving a life sentence? Her second husband, the late Leschelle, had been only slightly more fortunate. She had accused him of impotence and 'had ever after ill-treated him in such manner that the simplest account of it would outrage the hearing of any well-born person.' But for de Bray it was too late to change his mind. The unfortunate man had already exchanged his engagement vows. The nuptials were celebrated on 23 November 1573. It was a marriage which aroused some jealousy, to say the least, for fifteen days had not elapsed before certain ill-intentioned parties informed Marie d'Alvergne 'that the aforesaid De Bray was already supporting a wife by whom he had begotten several children before his marriage, and even that he did have carnal relations with women in several places.' Marie d'Alvergne immediately conveyed this to her daughter, 'the which did impress upon her a jealousy and low opinion of her husband.'

Subsequently, Marie de Corbie had several miscarriages as a result of the 'potions and medicaments which the aforesaid d'Alvergne, her mother, did make her consume, ostensibly to assist the child in her womb, or so she did claim.' Relentlessly, this pitiless harpy worked at destroying the love which her daughter still felt for her husband. She finally succeeded. 'Whereupon, they did consult as to the grounds on which they might bring a case for adultery. This path proving long and perilous, they did seek out a shorter one, to which the aforesaid d'Alvergne had formerly resorted, namely that of the dissolution of marriage on the grounds of impotence and frigidity.' From that moment, this incredible mother-in-law pursued her implacable hatred of the innocent De Bray until the verdict of annulment was finally declared.

It was again a mother-in-law, Madame de Soubise, mother of Catherine de Parthenay, whom the commentator of Bayle's *Dictionnaire* held responsible for the Quellenec case. This trial, he noted, 'ought in no sense to be attributed to Catherine de Parthenay, but to her mother. It was not the wife who did bring her husband before the law, but the mother-in-law that did litigate against her son-in-law.'

This accusation was not unwarranted. We have seen the relentless activity of Madame de Soubise in this sad affair. The 'Relation of what did take place in the matter of the dissolution of the marriage of Charles de Quellenec' is all the more unreliable in that it was drawn up at the request of the implacable mother-in-law. In it we can see the spider spinning the fatal web in which the Baron was to be caught. It was indeed she who pushed her daughter into this scandalous trial, as it was she who moved heaven and earth to solicit the intervention of those in the highest positions in the kingdoms of France and Navarre, and the condemnation of her son-in-law by the ministers of the Protestant religion. Catherine de Parthenay by contrast displayed the most remarkable discretion. By her obstinate silence, she seemed unwilling to repudiate either her husband or her mother, and she hesitated for a long time before formulating her accusation in public.

However, apart from the Quellenec case, in which the loud

and doubtless venomous interference by Madame de Soubise is indisputable, it is clear that many commentators exaggerated out of all proportion the role played by the mother-in-law in impotence trials. By placing the blame and infamy of a scandalous trial upon this scapegoat, they were attempting to preserve the halo of chastity which surrounded the very young girls who often got mixed up in these affairs. This apparently disinterested attachment to the ideal of youthful purity had profound psychological roots. It could not be undermined without destroying the intense belief in the young girl as a symbol of purity. Here the figure of Catherine de Parthenay, presented in Bayle's *Dictionnaire* as a saint, is an example. It was also, one may suspect, an essentially misogynistic reaction. The exaltation of one woman, distinguishing and isolating her from her fellows, constituted a mystification and a formidable weapon directed against the sex as a whole, by virtue of the insidious comparisons which it invited.

Moreover, laying the blame on the mother-in-law saved appearances. It allowed lawyers to flatter the self-esteem of their clients, arguing that their wives in fact loved them, and had it not been for their mothers-in-law . . . Finally, to condemn by a subtle strategy the conduct of the latter was to endorse the prejudices of a misogynistic public and judiciary, for whom the figure of the mother-in-law epitomised and incarnated all the defects of an abhorrent sex.

We have already mentioned cases in which the supposedly impotent man had fathered children, and this seems a strange paradox. How could the father of a family be accused of impotence? The rule *pater est quem nuptiae demonstrant* seemed to afford a precise answer to this question, by automatically legitimating any child born under the auspices of the conjugal union, whatever suspicions of adultery might weigh upon the mother. The Gautheu case, so often cited as a precedent by the jurists, served to enshrine this principle, which was not in fact supported by any canonical edict.

In 1643 (or 1639, according to which sources are used), Etienette Pipelier married Jean Gautheu. Three years later she had him summoned before the ecclesiastical court of Le Mans on a charge of impotence. The medical examination of his genitals proved inconclusive. If the marriage had not been consummated, said the report, the responsibility for this resided more with 'the aversions and impatience of the wife' than it did with the husband. In view of which, the ecclesiastical judge returned a verdict 'according to which he ordained that the husband and wife be sequestered a certain time to compose their thoughts to prayer, and by these prayers and other good works, to draw unto themselves the blessings of heaven.' Despite these noble words, Etienette Pipelier proceeded to indulge in 'unworthy practices' with a certain Mathieu Naïl. A few months passed, and she gave birth to a son who was baptised as 'the son of Mathieu Naïl and of Etienette Pipelier, born out of wedlock'. In the meantime, the ecclesiastical judge died. Etienette renewed her appeal for a dissolution with his successor, taking great care not to refer to her earlier appeal or to the birth of her child. This time, Gautheu, who had doubtless begun to appreciate the benefits of being single, declared himself to be impotent. He admitted 'to being in his own person that tomb of love of which spoke Atheneus, when he said that Venus had buried love in those chill and deathly herbs which he did term the food of the dead.' The marriage was declared 'null and dissolved'. Immediately afterwards, Pipelier and Naïl had their marriage banns published. But the latter's brother opposed the marriage and brought the case before the Paris High Court, citing the existence of a child as an accessory of abuse. On 5 July 1655 the court, by a verdict in accordance with the summing-up of the assistant public prosecutor Talon and with the rule *pater est quem*, declared 'that the dissolution

had been wrongfully and illegitimately initiated, conducted
and executed by the ecclesiastical judge of Le Mans, in view of
which the aforesaid Pipelier had been condemned to return to
the aforesaid Gautheu, her husband' and 'it has been forbidden
to the aforesaid Naïl and Pipelier to consort with each other on
pain of death.'

The rule *pater est quem* was not invoked solely in cases of
impotence, but also played a central role in settling disputes
between heirs.

In 1667 Monsieur de Mailly, father of two children, died.
The elder daughter of the deceased, together with two collaterals, attempted to exclude the younger son from the inheritance,
and they alleged that he was illegitimate. Their evidence was
based on a terrible confession made by a midwife called
Constantin shortly before she was hanged in 1660 for having
murdered several newly-born infants, the fruit of illegitimate
pregnancies. Fifteen years earlier, the De Mailly parents were
serving a prison sentence in the Fort l'Evêque. The mother,
who was then over fifty years old, was no longer able to have
children. She simulated a pregnancy and connived with the
midwife who, at an opportune moment, brought her a newly-
born infant which she had concealed in her apron after spirit-
ing it away from a cobbler's family. However, despite this
crucial testimony, when the case was tried in a hearing of the
Great Chamber the legitimacy of Nicolas de Mailly was confirmed by a verdict of 11 August 1667.

It seems that the rule *pater est quem* did in some cases admit
of exceptions. In his *Traité des Eunuques*, Ancillon gives an
account of a woman who, having accused her husband of impotence, was charged to explain the existence of her legitimate
child. In a jocular flight of oratory she confessed that 'she had
invited a stonemason that was at work in her house to see if he
could not do better than her husband . . . having lain her on
a chest that was nearby, he had done in but one attempt

that which her husband for all his pains had not been able to do this many a year.' Summoned at his wife's request, the husband admitted that 'he had lost one [testicle] through a gunshot, and the other through an illness'. The marriage was broken off and the wife married the natural father of her child.

This case, though it may have taken place, is of doubtful authenticity. The same cannot be said for the famous trial involving the Duc de Vendôme and the Duchesse d'Elbeuf, at the end of which the rule *pater est quem* found itself somewhat the worse for wear.

At the heart of this affair was the liaison between Gabrielle d'Estrée, the Duchesse de Beaufort, and Henri IV. In 1595, the beautiful Gabrielle bore a child, Cesar de Bourbon, duc de Vendome, who was immediately legitimised by the king. In 1651, fifty-two years after the death of Gabrielle d'Estrée, the Duchesse de Beaufort, Cesar de Bourbon's natural sister, lodged a request before the High Court of Paris attempting to exclude the Duc de Vendôme from 'the possession and enjoyment of all goods and property left by their mother.' Her reasons were simple. Gabrielle d'Estrée had been the lawful wife of the Duc de Beaufort when she gave birth to the Duc de Vendôme, the natural son of Henri IV. The circumstances of the birth annulled the letters of legitimation bestowed by the king, and as an adulterine son the duke was deprived of his rights to the succession.

The Duc de Vendôme answered these claims with two arguments.

Firstly, the marriage of the Duc de Liancourt and the Duchesse de Beaufort had been declared null 'in principle and from the outset' by a verdict of the diocesan ecclesiastical court. This decision was founded on 'the impotence of the said Sire de Liancourt; the which having occurred since his first marriage, by an uncommon accident as to which there exist authentic proofs, it did render him incapable of giving any legitimate consent to a legal action of this kind.'

Secondly, the Duc de Vendôme emphasised that he had been in possession of his present status for more than fifty years, which constituted a *de facto* validation.

The Duchesse de Beaufort next recalled the circumstances of the birth of the Duc de Vendôme, which occurred before any complaint had been lodged as to the impotence of the Duc de Liancourt. The child should therefore be considered either as the legitimate son of the Duc de Liancourt, by virtue of the rule *pater est quem*, or as the adulterine son of Henri IV. In either case, he would be excluded from the maternal succession. The argument was in vain. The court, by a ruling of 13 June 1651, declared the suit of the Duchesse de Beaufort to be inadmissible.

The exceptional character of this verdict should be emphasised, as well as the fact that it never set a precedent. Quite clearly the High Court had no choice in the matter. By submitting to the spirit of the rule *pater est quem* it would have both reversed a decision of the king of France and undermined a peer of the realm.

In the majority of cases, however, the rule was respected and applied without qualification – whence the efforts of several 'impotents' to guarantee the legitimacy of their marriage by arranging for their wife to conceive by extra-conjugal means.

One may ponder over the deeper meaning of this rule. Should it be regarded as a lifeline held out to certain impotent men by a lenient judge? It would be a mistake to believe this, for despite its mandatory character, the rule could not even exempt the 'impotent father' from legal proceedings. The fact that the latter were futile did not matter. The existence of the child confirmed the validity of the marriage, the final verdict was therefore known from the outset, yet the ecclesiastical judge never spared the accused from undergoing the humiliation of a gratuitous and cruel procedure.

On 18 May 1694, a man was summoned to appear before a court at the instigation of his wife, on a charge of impotence. In his defence he put forward an argument of considerable weight: was he not the legitimate father of a child baptised in his name? From the outset, the case was heard in his favour. Nevertheless, the unfortunate man was required to undergo an examination in due form. He refused to submit to this, arguing that the rule *pater est quem* was sufficiently clear concerning his status. The ecclesiastical judge appealed to the secular authorities for support, whereupon the man was thrown into prison and the questioning began. Several medical examinations followed. Because the Church judge was not satisfied with a single report, three were required. A dozen physicians and surgeons filed through the prisoner's cell. Soon, nobody was concerned with descriptions of his 'poor complexion' and 'pale face', but his genitals were the subject of the most detailed descriptions. These were 'found to be weak', 'the two testicles were flatulent', 'he has never had an ejaculation', 'he has no sexual appetite', 'he is injured in the neck of the bladder where are contained the prostate glands', 'a stone was discovered and removed the size of a pigeon's egg', and so on. The man no longer existed other than in these terms – he had become the property of the experts, who used and abused him as an object of experimentation. Analyses and verbal dissections succeeded each other at his bedside. The theories clashed, the reports thickened. The ecclesiastical judge delegated, summoned and reflected. When he finally asked the accused 'if he had been able ever to achieve carnal knowledge of the plaintiff', the former admitted 'that he was unable to ejaculate, nor had ever been able, having endeavoured without success on several occasions, both in the presence of the aforesaid E.P.D. and outside her presence, without being able to produce semen.'

This confession once extracted, the prosecutor, after holding consultations with nine theological doctors, pronounced the final verdict: 'All considered and the holy name of God having been invoked, as well as counsel heard, . . . We do hereby declare the aforementioned E.P.D. nonsuited in her request for an annulment of the marriage . . .'

The farce was over, but it had dragged on for twenty-two months.

Ultimately, the strict application of the rule *pater est quem* was motivated less by humanitarian principles than by social imperatives. 'It is a law that binds the family,' wrote the jurist Blondeau. 'It is an axiom of peace and concord for a husband reputed to be a father, for a wife that has become a mother, and for all relatives that are concerned about their succession. Regarding these, the rule is a proof, and is moreover endorsed by reason.'

Theologians and lawyers could easily overwhelm an impotent man who was solitary, isolated, marginal. But they could not undermine a father without gravely endangering the social system which they were pledged to defend and which was founded upon the institution of the family.

6

Attack and defence

When a request for annulment on the grounds of impotence appeared on the desk of an ecclesiastical judge, a cumbersome administrative machinery was set in motion. Cases of bigamy, rape or clandestine marriage could be settled by concrete evidence or incontrovertible testimony. Impotence on the other hand did not leap to the eye, but was a hidden disorder, an indiscernible evil which often lurked behind the most flattering appearances. Impotence was presumed rather than proven, and not even the most subtle reasoning could reach conclusions which were other than uncertain. It therefore became a point of honour to leave nothing to chance in the preliminary procedures. 'As impotence does involve the matter of a holy sacrament,' wrote Bouhier, 'common sense demands that the judge proceed with extreme circumspection, all the more so in that he can be so easily deceived, because of the uncertainty attending those proofs which can be furnished on such occasions.'

Faced with this complexity, the procedural structures multiplied and their methods varied increasingly. The element of uncertainty was providential, for it in fact gave lawyers and physicians a free rein. With a clear conscience they could acquire privileged access to all that was concealed from ordinary mortals by the dictates of modesty.

It seems appropriate at this point to say something of the litigants themselves. By definition, the average age and socio-professional background of the protagonists in impotence trials might seem easier to define than their underlying motives or psychological make-up. In fact, the printed sources are too heterogeneous and fragmentary to allow any rigorous statistical approach. The collection of archives for the ecclesiastical court of Paris during the period 1730–88 probably offers the most accurate picture, but we still have to rely to a large extent upon clues and approximations.

The average age of those accused of impotence is even more difficult to evaluate in that the records refer to a wide variety of ages within a very broad spectrum (Pierre Le Gros was only nineteen years old, whereas Jallot de Saint-Remi was sixty-five). The search for an average age moreover rests upon artificial assumptions, since the motives of the litigants differed fundamentally from one case to the next. Cases brought against old men were generally motivated by inheritance problems, whereas those ostensibly founded upon sexual frustration or desire were usually brought by very young women. Catherine de Parthenay was fourteen when she lodged her petition for annulment, Marie Magdeleine Mascranni was sixteen, Marie de Saint-Simon, the wife of the Marquis de Langey, and Martine Lebrun were both nineteen. In his twenty-third *plaidoyer*, Peleus discusses a girl of fifteen years who subjected her husband to trial by congress. In such cases the accused were also in general very young. De Gesvres was nineteen, Le Gros and De Langey were both twenty. This did not prevent the wives of older men from occasionally using the pretext of sexual desire: Jallot de Saint-Remi was sixty-five years old when his wife tried to subject him to trial by congress.

The sixteen impotence trials which emanated from the ecclesiastical court of Paris nevertheless indicate that, within the normal age limits (twenty-nine to fifty), the average age of men accused of impotence was forty, whereas the average age of 'supplicant' wives, within a larger normal age spectrum (sixteen to fifty), was around thirty.

The study of the socio-professional breakdown of litigants yields at least one certainty: the absence of any representation from the peasant population. Impotence trials were a privilege of the towns, and rural society was quite simply excluded. The indignation aroused by the behaviour of one country lass, Martine Lebrun, who inadvisedly entangled herself in this procedural labyrinth, underlines the exceptional nature of her initiative:

Here we do have a peasant girl [fulminated the lawyer Freteau] who wishes to distinguish herself from all others of her station . . .

By which act the respondent does plainly demonstrate to us an old and vulgar error that has held sway this many a year, namely the belief that innocence is especially to be found in rural parts . . .

On the other hand, an astonishing predominance of the nobility is revealed by an analysis of the collections of court records. Twenty per cent of all requests for annulment originated in the nobility, who represented only three per cent of the population. But although it is possible and even probable that nobles had a propensity to divorce on the grounds of impotence, here the printed sources should be treated with caution. Impotence trials enjoyed even more publicity than usual when the protagonists belonged to the upper classes. The prominence accorded to the nobility in the collections of court records is therefore not in itself surprising. Moreover, very often such families possessed the means to call upon the services of famous lawyers and to finance the compilation of factums which guaranteed their cases a resounding publicity. The archival sources were in fact far more discreet concerning the participation of the nobility in impotence trials.

The predominance of upper-class litigants was not entirely determined by financial reasons. While they were not negligible, the expenses incurred by the most basic type of proceedings were by no means ruinous. At the beginning of the eighteenth century, they were divided up as follows:

The Hubigneau Affair, 1700
No charge from us (the ecclesiastical judge); for each physician, 12

livres; for each surgeon, 9 livres; for each prosecutor, for two recesses, 12 livres; for the clerk of the court, 18 livres; for the concierge, 3 livres. (approximately one hundred livres in all)

At the end of the century, these fees had shown only a moderate increase:

The Chabrier Affair, 1783
Memorandum of the fees of the Officiality relative to one Jean Chabrier, wig-maker, accused by his wife of impotence:

– for the order of 29 March 1783 appointing physicians and surgeons to visit the said Chabrier	12 livres
– for the recess of the cross-examination on the same day	24 „
– for the recess for the various reports drawn up on 1 April	24 „
– for the fees paid to the physicians and surgeons	48 „
– for feeding the prisoner	6 „
– for paper	10 „
total:	124 livres

These rates applied to a case which was concluded in a fairly short time. The expenses could increase appreciably according to the number of juridical and forensic procedures involved.

Be that as it may, a trial could involve a quite different level of expense when the litigants enlisted famous lawyers, whose services and factums often ended by making holes in the family estate (De Bray, D'Argenton, De Gesvres, De Brosses, and so on).

Naturally, all legal costs were borne by the partner who was found guilty of impotence. In addition, it was the responsibility of an impotent husband to return the dowry and, in the majority of cases, to pay damages which sometimes came to a small fortune: 300 livres in the case of Rippert, 800 livres for the husband of Gabrielle de Mouchy, 2000 livres for one inhabitant of Castres.

But this was nothing in comparison to the moral opprobrium which was heaped upon a husband charged with impotence, and the mental or physical deprivation which threatened him if he could not free himself of his debts. 'Some have died of vexation for this reason', wrote Tagereau, 'others have lost their wits, and almost all have been ruined and made miserable.'

The extreme case is that of Poignant. Condemned as impotent in 1599 on the accusations of his wife, Catherine Martin, he was unable to repay the full amount of the dowry. He made a request to exercise the benefit of transfer, which the Paris High Court turned down in the belief that they were dealing with a charlatan. Thus he was imprisoned until such time as he could pay a sum which he was incapable of raising – in other words for life. His lawyer, Julien Peleus, painted a tragic picture of the situation:

What may it benefit his wife to see him die of hunger and frustration, in the mire and filth of prison, and together with him his closest relatives, on so vile a pretext as that of money? Is it not more urgent that this unfortunate should work in freedom so as to reach a state where he may acquit himself of his debts? [But] this woman or brute beast does turn a deaf ear to such reasoning, and wants only that he who had shared her bed should now be thrown into the gloom of mischance, that is to say into the public dungeons where, confined within high walls, he receives only the shadow of light that filters through the small grilles; where sits a hard-hearted porter who cannot be melted by the tears of a mother; and where the prisoners are covered in filth and their hands bound by chains.

In general, however, the costs of litigation in impotence trials did not make them the exclusive privilege of the very rich. In fact it was the liberal professions and the artisan class which figured more and more frequently in this kind of case. Printed and archival sources are agreed on this point. Physicians, barbers, surgeons, notaries, clerks of court, ushers, drapers, booksellers, grocers, gilders, wigmakers, saddlers, bakers and domestic servants all filed through the witness stand, united only by the fact that each had been summoned to answer the charge of his wife, after a period of cohabitation which varied from case to case.

The petition once lodged and the charge formulated, the chances of success were uncertain. However, what was certain even at this stage was that the judges would do everything in their power to extort the fullest testimony possible from the litigants. This is why a petition was never rejected out of hand, whatever its content. 'Under no conditions is an action halted,' wrote Claude Horry, 'in addition to which these petitions should be received favourably, for they do concern the salvation of the parties concerned, the which parties do lodge such pleas only in extremity, so that their good faith is to be relied upon ... For the marriage of an impotent is but an illusion of the holy sacrament, as would be that of a child.'

Doubtless the circumstances in which a petition was lodged and the marital background were taken into account. The length of time the couple had lived together prior to the lodging of the petition, or legal proceedings instituted by one of the partners against the other in the past were factors which sometimes affected the course of the case. But no hard and fast rules can be deduced.

According to Le Semelier, a wife who accused her husband of impotence within a short time of their marriage was less suspect than one who lodged a petition after several years of married life. A minimum of one or two months cohabitation after the nuptials was generally required by canon law before proceedings could be brought on the grounds of impotence according to 'De Frigidis et Maleficiatis'.

By a verdict of 28 July 1749, the ecclesiastical judge of Paris refused to grant a separation to Marie Louise Pochet and Jean Baptiste de La Hure, because they had been living together for twenty-seven years. That this delay in seeking a separation was extremely unusual can be seen from the fantastic contortions by which La Hure's counsel, Maître Thetion, attempted to justify his client:

The mystery, it has to be admitted, did take a long time to reveal itself. M. de La Hure, who was at the time deprived of that knowledge necessary to a married man, uninstructed in the secrets of the married state, yet more ignorant concerning Nature's whims and vagaries, did for a long time neglect to study or learn of those obstacles which he encountered in consummating his marriage. Night was wont to cover his efforts in the thickest darkness, and whether through consideration for his wife, through a misplaced modesty or shall we say weakness, he dared not to entrust his secret or enter into confidence with anybody else.

Thus did ten years elapse in this state of profoundest ignorance, after which a conversation with a midwife did finally enlighten him as to the situation of his wife.

The period of cohabitation was regarded as so solid an argument that it was sometimes invoked even in cases which were of an otherwise exemplary clarity. In 1649, the High Court of Paris had to give a ruling on appeal in the case of a wife who complained of her husband's sterility. From a juridical and canonical point of view, the suit was inadmissible, and the lawyers rejected it accordingly. But Lucien Soefve felt compelled to add that they 'did plead the case of the husband by invoking above all the fourteen years of his cohabitation with his wife.'

However, this trend was not uniform. Another commentator even cited the case of a man separated from his wife despite their having lived together for twelve years, and several jurists and theologians were careful to stress the silence of pontifical rulings concerning the time limit within which petitions for annulment were to be lodged.

Similarly, it is not clear whether the existence of a lawsuit initiated by the injured party, prior to the lodging of the petition and on a subject unrelated to impotence, had an appreciable effect upon the eventual outcome of the case. In a ruling of 12 June 1662, the High Court of Paris would seem to have answered this question in the affirmative. One year earlier, a certain De Gravière was judged impotent after a trial which took place before the courts of Tours and Lyons. His wife, Madame d'Espagne, remarried with complete peace of mind, whereupon the High Court of Paris, to which the case was submitted on appeal against an abusive practice, annulled this second marriage, prohibited 'the wife and her would-be second husband from consorting on pain of imprisonment', and referred the parties to the ecclesiastical judge of the archdiocese of Paris. The wife, by requesting a separation of goods and property shortly before her annulment suit, had implicitly recognised the validity of her marriage. Again, the consideration of specific case histories makes it impossible to generalise. It was not unusual for this same High Court to issue verdicts in different cases which contradicted each other.

If no general rule emerged concerning the effect of lawsuits engaged prior to the lodging of a petition for annulment, is it possible to determine more accurately the effect of a suit engaged after the charge of impotence was made?

Such cases were rare, but the problem deserves to be mentioned, for it surfaced dramatically during the Jean Costé affair. This case moreover had the distinction of involving a triple charge of maltreatment, impotence and adultery.

In 1631, an Orleans physician named Jean Costé married Madelaine Le Royer. Eighteen months later the household was shaken by a series of violent tremors. The drama centred around a presumptuous servant girl. Madelaine instituted proceedings with a view to obtaining a separation of goods and property. The provost of Orleans ruled that 'for a period of six months she was to be sequestered in the house of her mother, where Costé, her husband, could see her whenever it pleased him but was enjoined to put out of his house his domestic serving girl.' Costé's appeal was followed by a settlement between husband and wife. Shortly afterwards, the settlement was broken and the verdict of the provost quashed. Madelaine received orders to return to her husband. She refused. Costé lodged a suit, obtained a warrant for arrest and ordered his wife to be seized. The irrepressible Madelaine's reaction to this was characteristically biting: Costé found himself summoned to appear before the ecclesiastical judge of Orleans to answer a charge of impotence.

Appearing at this juncture, Madelaine's petition was obviously suspect. Despite this, it was received favourably. Costé challenged the court and lodged an appeal against abusive practice. Nonsuited by the High Court of Paris, he was handed over to the ecclesiastical judge. The case followed its course: cross-examinations, a medical examination . . . finally, trial by congress was ordered. At that moment the unfortunate Costé was thrown into prison for debt. He took advantage of his time by drafting a charge of adultery against his wife and obtained a 'decretal for the arrest of the aforesaid Royer, of a certain Rusignan and of several other persons . . .'

We may well ask ourselves, at this stage, which of the above charges was to be treated as prejudicial. As far as Madelaine Le Royer was concerned, the accusation of adultery was invalid by reason of the nullity of the marriage. The assistant public prosecutor Bignon was of the same opinion. The legal disability affecting Costé during the proceedings to determine his possible impotence had the effect of invalidating his accusation against his wife. At the same time, a charge of adultery could not be taken lightly, for it concerned public morals. Thus Jérôme Bignon turned down Costé's petition as inadmissible, but accepted the charge of adultery it contained and, taking the husband's place as a private party, entered the trial in the name of moral standards and on behalf of the public prosecutor. The impotence proceedings were now momentarily suspended to make way for an adultery case.

Thus, by means of a strategy steeped in hypocrisy, the judges avoided having to give up either of their victims. By giving a favourable reception to the accusation of adultery, they would have had implicitly to recognise the validity of the marriage and Costé's virility: the impotence trial would have slipped from their grasp. By rejecting the accusation outright, they would have had to exonerate Madelaine Le Royer and deprive themselves of the pleasure of acting as the champions of public morals. Repression won the day on both fronts.

The need to protect their social power and enlarge its scope explains the incredible voracity of ecclesiastical and secular judges. All petitions were thus accepted and treated with the greatest seriousness, whatever their content, the psychological and personal circumstances, the period of cohabitation or the juridical precedents. This opportunism could usually be sensed at the outset of a trial, and the subsequent course of events soon confirmed it.

In the meantime, the problem of the sequestration of the wife would have to be attended to, as the next step after her petition was lodged and accepted.

In theory, the question of whether the wife was to be sequestered or not involved the highest humanitarian considerations. It was a case of protecting the unhappy woman from the fury of a husband whose fatal flaw she had just revealed in public. In the majority of cases, the sequestration of the wife was favourably considered.

On 4 March 1610, the High Court of Paris, referred to on appeal by a husband deprived of his conjugal property, ruled that there was nothing improper in the decision of an ecclesiastical judge who had just ordered the sequestration of the wife in her father's house for the duration of the trial.

A ruling of the High Court of Grenoble followed suit on 4 September 1662. Here, moreover, we can discern an attempt on the part of the court – albeit a highly artificial attempt – to provoke a spirit of sexual competitiveness between Suzanne Auquier and Henry Fermier, by ordering that the wife

is to be sequestered for three months in the house of one of the relatives and friends of the parties, where the husband may come to see her day and night, and lie with her, and after this period the parties are to appear before the commissary, and will declare solemnly, each in the conspection of the other, whether the wife has been at any time known carnally by the husband. This being not the case, the parties will thereafter proceed to the medical visit and examination.

Five years later, the High Court of Provence returned a verdict contrary to the above, in the case of one Mademoiselle de Virail, who had been sequestered in a convent on the verbal orders of the bishop. It is true that here the sequestration occurred under different circumstances and in conditions whose legality was dubious. At the outset, the wife had expressed only a simple request for a physical separation and a separation of property on the grounds of 'the cruelties and ill-treatment of her husband, who did allegedly keep on the table four pistols, smoked tobacco and did other such things, though not to excess.' It was only later on 'and in passing that the aforesaid lady did request the court to be received with a view to proving the impotence of her husband.' The petition was accepted by the ecclesiastical judge, but was rejected by the High Court, which ruled 'that the permission accorded by the bishop to the nuns to remove the man's wife was improper.'

Far from any humanitarian considerations, the legal justification for sequestration ultimately rested on an openly misogynistic philosophy. For sequestration in the above instances clearly involved depositing temporarily in the hands of a third party an object whose ownership was in dispute. The husband had first of all to prove his ability to operate the object before he could reclaim it. In the eyes of the law, the title deed was acknowledged as valid only under these conditions. Moreover, an especially significant terminology surrounded this aspect of the woman as object. Boniface wrote in connection with the Auquier-Fermier case:

There is no right of possession, since there is no carnal cohabitation
. . . Fermier having been forced to admit before the whole court that
he had never known his wife carnally . . .
To request the restitution of a wife, the husband must prove that there
does exist a marriage in the sense of carnal cohabitation . . .
The wife having been known carnally, it is evident that her restitution
was bound to follow, since marriage had occurred.

The same coldness and cynicism is evident in the descriptions of the status of Mademoiselle de Virail, in response to her husband's loud demands that she be returned to him. The problem lay in deciding whether this 'husband despoiled of his wife should be reinstated in the possession and use of the latter . . . and she condemned to withdraw with him.'

One of the major issues at stake in the impotence trial was this notion of dispossession, for to deprive an individual of an object which was legally his was a serious breach of justice and of the established order.

After a petition had been lodged with the court, a preliminary enquiry might begin, and the question of evidence now became paramount. The demonstration of impotence relied upon a system which could offer no conclusive proof. Bouhier acknowledged this, and argued against the notion that uncertainty should therefore function as a prerogative of the law:

When a married woman is discovered lying with her gallant, it is treated as adultery, whether the crime has been committed or not. An act is declared groundless on the report of experts who have judged it to be thus. However, it may happen that they do mistake themselves, as many examples have shown. Certain unfortunates have even been condemned to the gallows on the merest circumstantial evidence, and often these circumstances or clues have served to condemn innocent victims.

The eminent jurist, whose attitude was one of gloomy resignation, salved his conscience by invoking human weakness and the spirit of the laws, which confer upon conjecture the status of proof.

This attitude was anticipated, a century and a half earlier, by Vincent Tagereau who pointed out, in a manner more critical than resigned, that 'canonists have taught several methods [for resolving impotence trials] that would better be termed assumptions than certain and assured evidence.'

Ultimately, Bouhier recognised, whether cynically or naively, that all dissolutions of marriage on the grounds of impotence rested exclusively upon assumption:

Since the Church has indicated several [assumptions], on which a marriage may be dissolved for reason of impotence, and since these rulings should be followed, we must not hesitate to conform to them.

It is true that the alternatives were always posed in dramatic terms: either dissolution or the profanation of a sacrament. According to Maître Begon, the choice should be made in favour 'of the party which has proof, although it be not demonstrative, and against the party which lacks proof, demonstrative or otherwise.'

Thus the marriage was confirmed only if the evidence against it was found to be in some sense suspect. Only as a very last resort was it regarded as 'better to risk confirming an invalid marriage than dissolving one that has been legitimately consummated.'

The recourse to a preliminary enquiry, though optional, was probably usual. But due to the secrecy in which it was held, it was rarely documented. Vincent Tagereau testified to the practice in the seventeenth century. It would take place 'on the premises where the husband lived', and its purpose was to ascertain 'whether he has not had relations with any other woman.' The conclusions of this enquiry generally placed the defendant at the centre of converging assumptions which by definition determined the subsequent course of the trial. At the same time, it allowed the investigator privileged access to the privacy of a household, 'the which,' notes Bouhier, 'would assuredly not be tolerated on any other pretext. In these cases however, no means should be spared to take the parties concerned by surprise.'

Pope Honorius III (1216–27) seems to have been the first to lend pontifical authority and prestige to this resolute and unwholesome intrusion of the Church into the private lives of its faithful. In a chapter entitled 'Litterae de Frigidis', he in fact approved the action of a judge who, 'to determine that one husband was in no sense falsely accused of impotence, had appointed the parish priest nearby to inquire whether the former had ever entertained relations with some other woman.'

The proof by *septima manus* reinforced the network of assumption and conjecture which formed the basis of the impotence trial. Its origins go back to Germanic criminal law, where the oath of litigating parties was valid only if supported by the testimony of seven relatives, friends or neighbours. When it was first introduced into Canon law, this practice was termed *rectum judicium*.

Judging by the accounts of Antoine Hotman and Vincent Tagereau, *septima manus* seems still to have been in force at the end of the sixteenth and beginning of the seventeenth centuries. The fate of litigants was thus linked to 'the affirmations of seven relatives or neighbours, who by saying yes do swear that the marriage has not been consummated.'

But even the law could not continue indefinitely to transgress common sense, and the *septima manus* finally fell into abeyance in the eighteenth century, 'given that relatives, not being party to what occurs in the marriage bed, could affirm nothing beyond their belief and suspicion that the marriage had not been consummated.'

The fall from grace of the *septima manus* provoked bitterness and nostalgia from the High Court judge Bouhier. After pointing out that the practice was still current in Italy and Spain, he remarked that 'there are but few families in which the absence of consummation does not soon come to the knowledge of those who see the couple regularly. Their faces, their speech, their behaviour, everything does instantly reveal the sad secret which must inevitably procure their divorce.'

It would have pleased Bouhier to learn that the proof by seven witnesses was to be rehabilitated during the nineteenth century, and that even today ecclesiastical magistrates have recourse to it when dealing with impotence.

The *septima manus* was the last of the preliminary procedures in impotence trials, after which the serious business began with the cross-examination of the litigants.

The cross-examination leads us to the heart of the trial and into the private life of the couple – to the very roots of discord. Here, the court's capacity to impose pain begins, though we are still far from the threshold of maximum suffering and dramatic intensity, which was reserved for the forensic proceedings. Nevertheless, the questions of the Church judge during the cross-examination had the cutting-edge of a scalpel, and the incisions made so carelessly into the already scarred past of the couple were clearly an exercise in mental torture.

The structure of the cross-examination often involved setting up a process of accusation which was often founded upon peripheral considerations. Before being tried for impotence, Pierre Randon was subjected to odious proceedings on a separate issue. A Protestant who had recently converted to Catholicism, he was first accused by the judge of having never truly renounced his earlier faith. Intrigue had motivated his actions. He was rarely seen in church, he scorned his Easter duties, he never went to confession. At repeated and inopportune moments, the cross-examination was punctuated with bizarre questions referring to his guilty and secret adherence to the reformed church.

A second pretext for incrimination was erected around a sordid affair which Pierre Randon was supposed to have skilfully organised to advance his own interests during his first marriage. Had he not forced his previous wife, Marie Rose Bonarme, to sign a document settling the income from a 'mutual gift' upon whichever partner outlived the other? And after contaminating his wife with that 'secret malady' which was the source of his impotence, had he not ended by abandoning her 'to the discretion of a certain Bellefond, a fat matron who was devoted to her'? And had the unfortunate wife not died shortly afterwards, struck down by an 'antimonial medicine' administered without proper supervision? To make things worse, Pierre Randon was supposed to have married his second wife, Marie-Catherine Maurroy, in the hope of reaping similar advantages. Buried beneath the mud of these accusations, the question of Randon's impotence surfaced only episodically during the cross-examination, and the ecclesiastical judge seemed primarily concerned with destroying the accused on the grounds of his supposed allegiance to Protestantism. The cross-examination of Catherine Maurroy, which was of a disarming brevity and leniency, would bear out this interpretation.

In other cases, niggling and ludicrous insinuations are to be found side by side with serious accusations. It is sufficient to mention the example of Jean Auffroy, who was formally required to explain why he got out of bed one night, around five in the morning, in his underclothes, to go into the courtyard, and why he returned, still in his underclothes, to go back to sleep beside his wife. 'I had heard a knock at the door,' was the defendant's reply.

However, in the majority of cases, impotence naturally

afforded the ideal pretext for accusation. An insurmountable prejudice hung over any individual submitted to a cross-examination. Resistance was futile; the questions fused into a single monotonous cry of denunciation. For how long had he known himself to be impotent? What was the origin of his impotence? What were the symptoms? Had he consulted a physician? Did he know he was impotent at the time of his marriage? Was he aware that he had profaned the sacrament? Admission did not put an end to the torture, for the ecclesiastical judge wanted to know everything about the evil afflicting the impotent husband. Relentlessly, and impelled by a kind of sadistic relish, he would ponder the smallest details. The same treatment was reserved for an impotent wife, as in the following case of an unfortunate woman who confessed to her incapacity. The judge ploughed on with ponderous insistence:

Enquired, as to whether the aforesaid impotence was natural or accidental, whence it originated and in what year.

Replied, that the impotence which could be said to afflict her did proceed from a fall that she had at the age of seventeen years, and which did cause a collapse of flesh inside her womb, projecting as far as the exterior of her sex such as to block the entry, and from which she does suffer great external pains such as to prevent her even from holding her urine.

Enquired, as to whether the disorder was continuous.

Replied, that she is never out of pain and that the fleshy protuberance does never retract.

Enquired, as to whether the aforesaid D, her husband, had never made natural intromission into her.

Replied, that no, or the little that he had managed was achieved at the cost of such pain on her part that she could not support him inside her . . .

The ecclesiastical judges were never satisfied with incrimination, and insisted always upon learning as much as possible of the public and private lives of the couple. How did they meet? Through whom? Where was the marriage solemnised and celebrated? But the sphere of their activity which received the most prolonged attention was, naturally, that of the bed-chamber, through which the following learned theologian stalks as if through conquered territory:

Enquired, if it were not true that for a year, since the wedding day itself, he had made no advances to the aforesaid Ch. such as are customary between man and wife.

Enquired, if he had not employed his fingers to tear and make all bloody the private parts of the plaintiff.

Enquired, if it were not true that the marriage being solemnised, the aforesaid Louis Henry Besnard, desirous of advancing upon his wife, had been unable to consummate the marriage because of an involuntary ejaculation.

Enquired, if it were not true that he essayed for the first time on the fourteenth night after the marriage, and that having exhausted his efforts was obliged to withdraw.

Enquired, if it were not true that his semen was misdirected away from the appropriate orifice and scattered round about.

Faced with such questioning, what strategies could the accused adopt?

These cross-examinations do not only enlighten us as to the mentality of the judges; they also throw a harsh light upon the psychology of the couples.

For the accused man, any charge of impotence was in a sense unbearable. Held as ransom to this ancient myth of virility which so few civilisations have been able to exorcise, he defended himself as he could. Most often, this meant adopting a flexible system of defence, taking care not to claim perfect virility. Thus he would admit openly that the marriage had not been consummated on the wedding night, as a simple tactical retreat intended to make his subsequent statements more credible, and perhaps to insinuate that an initial and passing weakness on his part must have inadvertently sown the seed of his wife's future accusations of impotence.

Henry de Hou . . . acknowledged that a painful illness had imposed upon him a regime of strict continence. 'He was pulmonic and did often spit blood at this time.' He had therefore resisted his wife's attentions by simulating deep sleep. Subsequently, everything reverted to normal.

The Marquis de Gesvres had indigestion through having eaten an eel pie.

Pierre Randon had caught a chill, so that his whole body trembled. He had moreover discovered on his bride's body the signs of childbirth, which had thrown him into a fury. Under such circumstances, the consummation of the nuptials was postponed till later.

Jean Auffroy had told Marie Boutelouys that the physician who was to operate upon him in six weeks' time had forbidden him to have any sexual relations until after the operation.

Claude Chevalier had broken two ribs on his wedding day, by carrying a man who had fallen ill in his tavern.

Sometimes, the excuse was made as an attack, implicating a wife who deliberately refused any attempts at consummation.

Thus a certain F.D.B. 'had not wished to consummate the marriage, placing two pillows beneath her head so as to make difficulties for the aforesaid Sire A. and to ward off his advances.'

Hubigneau asserted that his wife, Anne Gabrielle de La Motte, 'had refused to perform her conjugal duty time after time, by adopting postures which did make it impossible for him to advance upon her.'

Jean Sturm and Marie Renard had shared the same bed for only thirty-eight nights in all. But, 'whenever he wished to advance upon her, take her by the hand and perform those caresses that a husband does owe to his wife, she would rebuff him with indignation, saying: "Keep away, I feel unwell, do you not know me still" and other tirades of this kind, capable of freezing the most robust husband and the strongest temperament.'

An allegation supported by concrete proof was more unusual, and these tended to rest upon tenuous arguments. The Marquis de Gesvres, for example, claimed that the domestic servants and the laundresses had seen the wedding sheets stained with blood, and that this was irrefutable proof of consummation.

In desperation, a reference to a pregnancy was likely to be taken more seriously:

Marie Magdeleine Mascranni supposedly had a miscarriage as a result of a fall. She was even supposed to have declared at the time: 'Were I to become pregnant, it would upset all my plans.'

According to Nicolas Sene, Catherine Chardon announced repeatedly and to several people that she thought herself pregnant.

Pierre Randon spoke of a still-born child by his first wife.

The accusatory strategy of the opposing party also depended upon a limited number of favourite themes, foremost among which was the obliging narrative of the impotent husband's perverse lechery:

Randon 'did desire to fondle his wife's body with impure caresses that bore little relation to the consummation of a marriage.' To which he replied that he had 'all rights over the body of his wife, and that he had wished to see her all naked.'

The judge Charles Adhemet asked Claude Chevalier 'if it were not true that, to excite himself the more he was often wont to place Mademoiselle Blanchet naked before his eyes, and to fondle her with his fingers, without this procuring the slightest effect or benefit.'

More innocently, the Marquis de Gesvres would pass entire nights next to his wife, tirelessly lavishing 'new protestations of his undying love upon her, and embracing her lovingly, but without arriving any nearer to a consummation of the marriage.' After the candid Madame de Gesvres had made, in Maître Begon's words, 'some progress in the Theory', the

Marquis 'did hide himself in his night-shirt' and took her by the hands lest, by some more uncompromising gesture, she might demand more of him.

The impotent husband was sometimes accused of having attempted to engage the services of some womaniser capable of deflowering his wife and providing him with a child:

After Jean Auffroy confessed his impotence to Marie Boutelouys, he was supposed to have said that 'if she was desirous to bear children, as he knew that she liked them, she could have someone visit her; he would not find this bad, but on the contrary, he would be pleased to have a child.'

For several months, Nicolas Sene was said to have imposed on his wife the presence of a stranger under the conjugal roof, 'who slept in a bed in the passageway of her chamber. This was not all, for the intruder would dress and undress before her eyes. One morning, she did find him in her bed.' According to the husband, this man was in fact merely a cousin of his wife, who lived in the house at the request of his wife's parents. Out of hospitality, he had given him his bed one night, as the cousin's bed had been 'wetted by a child.'

Such accusations indicated a profound unease, an irrevocable incompatibility. At the heart of this conjugal hell, physical violence was naturally unleashed in the wake of verbal violence.

Thus the wife referred to in accounts as F.D.B. was accused of having maltreated her husband, L.H.A. She declared that 'when she saw him, she believed she was looking at the Devil; that she hated him and would hate him always.' The unfortunate man, 'wishing one day to be intimate with her, she had squeezed his genital parts with such force and violence that he thought he was dying, having instantly lost all respiration . . . On several other occasions, she had bitten him, scratched him and tried to strangle him, all simply to avoid suffering his advances . . .' In the course of a journey to Narbonne, 'she had abused him . . . saying outrageous insults, striking him, maltreating him . . . she did strike him in the face with her fist . . . she scratched him in fury and one day she did bring a candle to his face and wig . . . She told him that she would stab him, one day, and did run to take a sword . . . While in Narbonne she did receive in her chamber almost every day a young man from Païs, with whom she would continue in conversation till two or three hours after midnight . . .'

In order to prevent word of his impotence from spreading, the Marquis de Gesvres exiled his wife to the country. Banished to 'this unwholesome solitude', she contracted 'nettle-rash, smallpox, measles and fever together with an infinity of alarming symptoms such as the vapours and fainting fits.' The Marquis then decided upon an obnoxious form of blackmail. He tried to negotiate her return in exchange for a letter stating that the marriage had been consummated. When she finally returned to Paris, after ten months, she was 'almost dying'.

Out of frustration, Nicolas Sene 'once in the night did kick his wife out of bed all naked onto the floor.' In this sorry state, 'half dead', she begged him to seek the aid of her relatives, which he refused. On another occasion, he gave her a potion, and 'after she had taken it, she did find her throat and stomach all afire.'

Again, possessed by a sudden fury, Randon struck his wife 'with his fist such as to knock out a tooth.'

The La Hure-Pochet affair draws an even more sordid picture. A peaceable tailor, La Hure found himself increasingly confronted by his wife's unstable character. In the cross-examination he was to paint a Dantesque picture of their life together. We see her wandering in the countryside without food or drink, attempting to put an end to her days by throwing herself into a well where the water was only thirty centimetres deep, knocking her head against walls. Moreover, she would rouse up the neighbourhood, rushing around the tradesmen and describing her husband as a man crippled by debts. Thus the unfortunate man found his credit stopped, himself on the verge of ruin, and his house reduced to 'an abode of sorrow and despair.'

In turn, Marie Louise Pochet delivered her version of their misery. She was resigned to her position as a wife, and impotent, admittedly, but only through the fault of a husband who had never made advances to her. In her own house, La Hure had imposed on her the presence of his mistress, Jeanne Tintelin, and openly displayed their relationship. 'Through her licentious attentions and servility,' wrote Maître Coquereau, 'this former servant girl did teach him to prefer the novelties of twenty-one-year-old Hagar to the constant and loving attachment of forty-five-year-old Sarah.' Jeanne Tintelin gave birth to a child, and soon the two lovers began conspiring to get rid of Marie Louise Pochet. They passed her off as insane, and had her confined in a lunatic asylum on two occasions.

However, violence was not the only manifestation of conjugal hell which was revealed in cross-examinations. Incompatibility sometimes originated in illnesses whose symptoms were especially repugnant. Louis-Henri Bénard had a face and body covered in sores 'deriving from those of scrofula'. He had hidden them more or less effectively prior to his marriage by attributing them to 'a heated liver', and by concealing his hands in gloves. But on the wedding night his mask fell — literally. After a miserable attempt at consummation, 'his skin became attached and as it were glued to that of the aforesaid Lemaître girl, through the suppurations of the sores which covered his body.' Soon, Bénard, his wife, the bed-curtains and the sheets were all inextricably joined in a suppurating mass:

After his advances, the bed-linen became stuck to the aforesaid Lemaître girl as well as to himself, through the said suppuration of humours which did issue from his scabby sores . . . Three weeks and even one month after the wedding night, the effects of his illness were so considerable that each morning when rising, his nightshirt was attached to the sheets and to his skin as well as the night table.

By now Anne Lemaître was infected, and blossomed in turn. Moreover, the exhalations which emanated from the bed each night caused her to have bouts of nausea and vomiting. The windows had to be left open throughout the winter. As for Bénard, he had begun playing out a strange comedy. He would conceal his dirty linen in a locked cabinet prior to taking it, once a week and in great secrecy, to his personal laundress. In these circumstances impotence, one of the signs of which was 'involuntary ejaculation, occasioned here by that same illness which had drained his blood of its vigour', could be alleged only as a subsidiary reason for separation.

Judges were well aware that a straightforward incompatibility of temperament or some other problem of a non-sexual nature could in certain cases provoke an accusation of impotence. This was why they made a point of setting up a forensic system of control.

7

The science of misogyny

The legal procedures for dissolution of marriage on the grounds of impotence afforded judges the right of unlimited inquiry into the private life of the individual. By assigning to experts the responsibility for pronouncing on virility or impotence, virginity or defloration, the ecclesiastical courts delegated to doctors, surgeons and midwives an absolute right to investigate the bodies of the couple involved in a dispute. Inspection of the genitals, proof of erection and trial by congress obviously constituted a respectable front for the play of an unacknowledged libido and exacerbated voyeurism. The execution of these procedures and the style of the experts' reports leave no doubt on the matter.

The experts' knowledge and the judges' skill, however, offered no final solutions. Uncertainty and speculation were the outcome of impotence proceedings. The physicians, jurists and the Church abdicated responsibility and, once again, Bouhier asserts a clear conscience on the matter:

While the Church exhorts the judges to employ scrupulous circumspection in this sort of case, it does not, however, prohibit their waiting before pronouncing a verdict on the dissolution of the marriage until complete certainty of the husband's impotence exists, because, while there are cases in which it may be perfectly well proven, there are others in which it is so beclouded that it may only be proved by supposition.

Physical examinations of both men and women were an important element in many of the impotence cases recorded. Accounts exist of the examination of the genitals in a variety of circumstances and, unlike trial by congress, there is no doubt that the practice was universal and widespread in time and place.

It was not a new phenomenon. The Romans certainly used it to assess the nubility of the young as part of a prenuptial examination. According to Bayle, however, in the sixth century Justinian 'could no longer suffer that the puberty of the male be decided by inspection of the parts of shame. He set the age at fourteen, be they vigorous or not, regarding the custom hitherto as a very dishonest practice.'

Sébastien Roulliard refers to the testimony of Amien Marcellin, however, stating that in the fourth century, examination of the genitals as part of an impotence trial already existed in the Eastern Empire. The text cited by him concerns the complaint addressed by a husband to the Patriarch of Constantinople regarding his wife's impotence. The case was quite unique, even in the eyes of the Byzantines:

The Patriarch, astounded by a complaint on such a novel theme, wished solemnly to acquaint himself thereof, accompanied by the clergy, his suffragans and diocesans, on whose counsel he ordered that she be examined by the principal doctors of the city. Being found to be too narrow on inspection, the marriage was declared never to have occurred.

In the West, systematic recourse to examination of the genitals in disputes only really became common in the twelfth century, and was institutionalised a century later by Innocent III.

A document from this period discusses it, indeed, as common practice:

Any woman that desires severance or separation from her husband because he cannot be of company to her flesh or cannot deflower her must be examined.

Well before the sixteenth century, these examinations became widespread in Europe, and Bouhier states that 'this formality is practised in all the ecclesiastical courts not only of Italy, Spain and of the Low Countries but also of this Realm.'

The 'visit' (as such medical examinations were known) was not, however, restricted to impotence trials. It occurred in cases of defamation, rape, premarital defloration and even of bestiality. It was by this means that the Virgin Mary and Joan of Arc came to embody virginity in its noblest form. Sébastien Roulliard recalls that an examination of Mary's natural parts was ordered by the Sanhedrin of the High Priest, 'to know if she had remained a maid and if our Lord her son should be raised to the ranks of the High Priesthood.' When Joan of Arc presented herself to Charles VIII charged with a divine mission, she claimed to be a holy woman by reason of her virginity. The midwives who examined her on the King's orders confirmed her virginity.

In another area, a premarital examination perhaps allowed the nubility of adolescent girls destined for a princely marriage to be assessed. The chronicler Froissart wrote: 'It is the custom in France that any maid as the daughter of a noble lord agrees to be contemplated and appraised entirely naked by ladies, to know whether she be suited and formed to bear child.'

In cases of defamation, examination of the genitals became of major importance. It was by such means that the case of the Sabbath of Place Maubert came to a happy conclusion.

In 1560, several Protestant meetings took place in Paris by night. Innumerable calumnies were willingly circulated on this subject by Catholics. Alarmed by the persistence of public rumours, Catherine de Médicis instructed the High Court judge of Saint-André to investigate. Two children heard as witnesses stated that:

In the Place Maubert, in the house of a lawyer named Boulard, there were held several assemblies of Lutherans, at one of which on the Thursday before Easter assembled a great number of men, women and maids around midnight when, having preached, made the Sabbath and eaten a pig in lieu of the paschal lamb, and the lamp having been extinguished, each did couple with his mate, and, among other women, the witnesses did recognise the aforementioned lawyer's wife and two of his beautiful young daughters, one of whom, coming upon one of these, was known by him twice or thrice.

The case was brought to law, but a genital examination cleared the two young girls of any suspicion.

A host of petty, everyday denunciations made these examinations necessary. The case of a priest accused of hermaphroditism by one of his colleagues and found innocent upon examination has already been cited. The lawyer Le Noble speaks of another priest accused by a curate of being the lover of his sister-in-law and the father of his 'nephews'. To clear his name, the unfortunate man declared himself impotent and demanded an examination of his genitals.

Nuns seem to have attracted slanderous rumours even more often than priests and, in spite of the uncertainties of the method, a physical examination doubtless settled more than one such case.

The benefit of the examination was also extended to the victims of abduction. 'What other course is there for honest maids,' asks Bouhier, 'that have had the misfortune to be abducted against their will and who desire to prove consummation of the rape, but to allow the inspection of their persons?'

Premarital consummation was also confirmed or disproven by examination of the genitals. Hercules Bouvard asked for the hand of Marie Heard, stating that he had carnal knowledge of her not 'out of lewdness' but to ward off 'noueurs d'aiguillettes, which he had previously experienced to his great displeasure.' On 20 August 1604 the High Court of Paris decided to rule on this case in accordance with the conclusions of the examination report.

Above all, however, it was the accusations of rape brought before the attention of the civil lieutenant that required a systematic and scrupulous examination of the alleged victim.

This procedure had already been applied in the thirteenth century, as shown by a document cited above, which stipulates that the 'examination must be carried out by seven widows or married women worthy of trust, so that defloration may be proven if appropriate.' Four centuries later, one report of rape cited by Dr Venette lists a physical inspection of the victim that extended to the nipples, pubic hair, the vagina, the clitoris, the cervix, the vulva and the hymen.

Finally, it seems that examinations of virginity were carried out in certain cases of suspected bestiality. During the examination of Claudine Culam, who was 'accused of having had carnal copulation with a dog', the attitude of the 'seducer' was to say the least ambiguous. Indeed, 'it did put up a resistance and would not cease from raising with its muzzle the skirts of the Culam woman', from which the pious judges concluded that 'it was quite shameful to suffer one's skirts to be lifted thus, being thereby so indecently uncovered before all and sundry.'

The widespread practice of these apparently respectable examinations did, however, inevitably raise serious legal and moral problems.

From the end of the sixteenth century, genital examinations of women were at the centre of an unresolved and consistently impassioned polemic. The detractors, jurists or physicians, claimed that such examinations undermined notions of decency, and were flagrantly inconclusive. Paradoxically, examinations of the genitals of a man caused no embarrassment. The proof of erection, which constituted a high point of obscenity, evinced only mild reactions, usually from interested parties. The greatest outcry concerned the undressing of women, which provoked a prudish indignation in which inhibition was combined with a certain morose excitement. It also provoked the annoying but highly significant question: could nudity, the shameful and disastrous attribute of original sin, be reconciled with the ideal of evangelical purity which ought to inspire the judges of the Church?

The shameful parts of woman, it must be said, exerted a troubled fascination over the participants of this debate and inspired a host of baroque commentaries.

Thus Vincent Tagereau: 'The bodies of drowned men are always discovered on their backs, facing upwards. Those of women, on the other hand, are found on their front, face down, as if Nature, considerate of their honour, would hide that in them which may not honestly be seen.' For Tagereau, the lessons of history merited the same attention as those of nature. 'This stripping,' he continues, 'was formerly a sort of punishment for adulterous women.'

In the same spirit, Anne Robert becomes indignant that 'young maids, that one supposes to be virgins, not only willingly endure, but do ask insistently that an exhibition be ordered of those parts of shame which the persecutors of Christians and enemies of Religion do likewise order for the greater martyrdom and dishonour of the faithful whom they punish.'

Moreover, undressing a woman provoked the senses and roused the basest instincts. 'Can it be,' asks Anne Robert, 'that there is anything more lascivious, that arouses the senses and excites lewdness more, than uncovering those secret parts of the body which Nature itself has hidden, or revealing those crude and uncontrived members which self-discipline and shame have hidden beneath movements and aspirations to holiness?'

Drawing upon the authority of Saint Augustine, Saint Ambrose and Saint Cyprian, opponents of the examination recalled that this test had no basis in Canon law. The position of Saint Ambrose was especially clear. He formally condemned the bishop of Verona, Syagrius, who had ordered an examination of a nun accused by public rumour of giving birth to a child in secret and then having it killed. When questioned on the case of a nun accused of sexual incontinence, Saint Cyprian showed the same firmness of attitude.

Thus the example of the Church fathers ought to have inspired Christians. It was, however, rare that an ecclesiastical judge, though responsible for the examination, was mentioned by name. The 'customs of the time', the 'corruptions of this age' and even the woman in question were readily cited instead, the latter being the particular object of attention for opponents of the examination. 'She that complains of her husband's impotence and, in order to achieve separation, does permit men to uncover her, to see and handle those parts which Nature would have her hide,' wrote Tagereau, 'must be considered immodest and shameless.'

In less colourful language, Héricourt, two centuries later, expressed the same sentiment: 'Certain women have asked that their husbands be judged impotent by inspection of their own person . . . but such a request is itself unbecoming on the lips of a lady of honour.' During the same period, the theologian Sainte-Beuve, in a spirit of evangelical purity, called for the abolition of 'so shameful and dishonest a practice'. In his opinion, spouses were to be reconciled by undergoing a three-year period of cohabitation, in accordance with the spirit of the early Church. At the end of this test, the judge would accept the declarations of the couple made under oath.

The shame which it inspired was not the only criticism levelled against the examination. The uncertainty of its conclusions was another argument for its abolition. Virginity was not as easy to determine as some believed.

At the heart of the impotence trial, then, the secular problem of the hymen was posed in dramatic terms. At the end of the sixteenth century, Dr Joubert wrote that 'this matter is of great importance for the honour or dishonour of maids, for the dissolution of marriage contracted with an impotent, frigid or bewitched person, and for the censure or absolution of one accused of forcible rape.'

Whether a figment of the imagination or not, the hymen inspired a rich poetic vein which had lain dormant in magistrates and physicians during the sixteenth and seventeenth centuries. The myths which surrounded it are not without interest, for they burgeoned in the service of the controversy over the examinations of the genitals.

A myth for some, a reality for others, this hypothetical membrane nevertheless persisted as a universally powerful symbol. Until the end of the seventeenth century, it elicited from the most austere authors a streak of tenderness and a stream of metaphors tinged with the breath of spring. Was woman not the earth and the womb its most delicate part? In such a universe, the hymen, symbol of an earth primed to yield fruit, was the natural repository of the virtues and freshness of spring. It was a 'flower', a 'flower of virginity' (Tagereau, Severin Pineau). Once this 'flower of maidenhead' was 'plucked', the youthful virgin who 'has allowed master mole to burrow within' (Duval) was 'deflowered'. In the eyes of Dr Venette, who composed a resonant panegyric to virginity,

it is a beautiful flower conserved in a garden that is walled on all sides. No implement has harmed it by cultivating it. A kind breeze wafts it, a temperate clime maintains it and a gentle rain does water it and make it grow. Every youth desires it passionately, but it is no sooner plucked than despised.

Again, the hymen was the tangible mark of purity, a 'token' and a 'seal' (Tagereau, Anne Robert). It was the 'ornament of manners, the holiness of the sexes, the wealth of modesty, the bread of families, and the source of the most blessed friendships' (Venette). Against the assaults of concupiscence this 'Lady in the middle' held vigilant watch. She guarded the 'virginal cloister', kept 'the watch on virginity' (Du Laurens) and acted as a 'hedge' or 'rampart' (Joubert).

The sentimental attachment to the hymen arose out of deep-seated aspirations. The universal respect which surrounded virgins has already been discussed. The cult of the mythical integument called the hymen, an object of verbal devotion and adulation even on the part of sceptics, was the logical consequence of this respect. The need to believe in an ideal of purity and chastity was too strongly rooted in the structures of consciousness for rationalism or anatomical observation to upset its powerful and symbolic functions. Moreover, the hymen fetish was based on an age-old tradition, the geographical breadth of whose manifestations is quite remarkable.

The exhibition of nuptial sheets stained with virgin blood illustrates another aspect of the myth. The extension of this Biblically-inspired practice to the Mediterranean gave rise to florid and occasionally nostalgic descriptions. These were often accompanied by a mise-en-scène which happily combined exhibitionism and curiosity. Thus in the kingdom of Fez, the newly-weds were locked in one room while their guests waited in the adjacent one. Only when the couple managed to produce a bloodstained sheet could the feast commence. Otherwise, the wife 'is returned by the husband to her father and mother, who derive great shame therefrom, while the guests do return home on an empty stomach.'

According to another account, 'the Spaniards, that are great observers of ceremony, on the day following the wedding do have matrons show the sheets of the nuptial bed in public with great acclaim, to parade the stains of defloration, crying out all the while from a window: *Virgen la tenemos.*' In the kingdom of Naples, the young bride was subjected to the same ordeal, and it is not certain that this tradition, which was still referred to in the eighteenth century, has completely disappeared even today.

To the seventeenth-century observer, these practices were

by no means exotic. Joubert, Duval and Venette mention equally colourful procedures used by midwives to determine whether the hymen was intact. There were some fifteen signs of 'violation' that were generally recognised. In addition to these there were other methods of appraisal which, in spite of their purely subjective nature, could be taken, if not as evidence, then at least as assumptions in certain impotence trials.

Virgins turn into discomfited, morose women, 'because, being deflowered, even though this be honestly done and by marriage, the girl has a subdued and shameful aspect, a tender and bashful, sad look in her eye. Blushes then do rise to her cheek when she sees intimates of her family.' In Duval's description, virginity sparkles with joy and health:

The eyes look beauteous with a naive gaiety in the maid. But after that flower of maidenhead has been plucked, the white of the conjunctive membrane that is in the eye does appear lustreless and the gaze sadder than before . . .

The tip of the nose, that is fleshier in the maid, does appear as gaunt and cloven in she who has lost her maidenhead . . .

When the maid begins to enjoy the embraces of a man, her voice, that previously rang out clear, does begin to sound deep and harsh . . .

The maid who in full health had rejoiced in her maidenhead, when agitated by the efforts of her cabinet being unlocked, will exhibit some disdain for meats and is even caught unawares by nausea and vomitings.

Some experiments were employed to confirm the above diagnoses:

Administer to her a little pounded wood of aloes to drink or eat. If a maid, she will piss incontinently.

With a thread, measure the girth of the neck and then from the chin to the top of the head. If the measures are equal, she is a maid. If the neck be larger, she is corrupted.

The maid pisses more clearly and finely than another, because her parts are tighter and strait to the outer edge, making her piss firmer and farther.

Most scholars, however, were not moved or blinded by a terminology so heavily laced with fantasy. They mistrusted such superstitious wedding ceremonies. As for the so-called signs of virginity, they referred to them only in banter and generally treated the hymen with scepticism.

The persistence of the myth of the hymen, and its currency in learned circles right up to and during the eighteenth century, is therefore surprising, particularly since there is no doubt as to the scepticism of anatomists at the end of the sixteenth century. Some, it is true, admitted the existence of a film at the opening of the cervix. In a treatise published in 1598 under the title *De integritatis et corruptionis virginum notis*, the surgeon Séverin Pineau even claimed that the hymen was not composed of a single membrane, but of four small pieces of flesh which meet, thereby hermetically sealing the 'passage of modesty'.

For others, this incongruous medley of different interpretations was no more than 'pure daydream', 'poetic fiction' and 'a heap of follies'. Ambroise Paré willingly admitted 'that in twenty thousand virgins, this pellicule or film is not to be found', and its extremely rare occurrence in the form of an 'unnatural fold' he linked to an organic defect. The illustrious surgeon never detected the slightest trace of it in the course of his dissections of young girls.

The hymen was similarly invisible to the keen eye of Du Laurens, who 'diligently considered (and probed) girls born before time, others of only three months, and others of three, four, six and seven years.' Moreover, this surgeon conducted a very strange experiment on the genitals of a young girl:

If, using a drinking straw, you fill the outer parts of the passage of shame with wind, the whole cervix will be observed to dilate and open up, so that the road lies open from the external orifice, termed the vulva, all the way to the inner entrance to the womb.

The discharge of blood accompanying the first sexual relations was not to be confused with the rupture of a non-existent membrane. Paré explained it as being due to small blood vessels bursting under the strain of the first intromission. Occasionally, it was 'unevennesses of the cervix' which, according to him, caused the bleeding.

As for the tests of virginity, these were fittingly part of the arsenal of untrained midwives. The experiments of these 'good wives' were 'things so vain and uncertain, that one must by no means put one's trust therein.' For nothing could be deduced from the dilation of the open vagina of a virgin 'who on occasion may have put her finger good and deep into the cervix because of some itch she might have there.' On the contrary, such a virgin was blessed with 'a channel comfortably dilated and easily stretched because of its natural breadth and softness.' Whereas 'another, in whom some churl may have forayed with his little tool, will have a channel that is tight by nature and will be held to be a maid.' 'Tousled' (flattened) pubic hair signified nothing, 'because, since maids and ladies have learned to ride in the Italian style, with the knee braced against the saddle bow, their hair is not so well ordered, being somewhat tousled, and the *mons* is flatter in form than on other females that ride with their thighs held close together.'

Some observers were not content to refute the myth of the hymen in purely anatomical terms. Thus the surgeon Guillemeau shifted the debate into the philosophical realm, musing on the purpose of the hymen:

Nature does nothing in vain, but creates all for a certain end, use and intention. Now, what employment could She argue for this part, why must it have been woven and placed in this spot by Nature: is it to enhance the pleasures of Venus? Is it to defend the womb against the cold or other injury?

During the same period, the jurists Anne Robert and Tagereau expressed an identical opinion. In their view, the hymen did not exist. Solomon's proverb, constantly quoted by the authors, was considered to be the last word on the subject: Solomon said that are four things that surpass human understanding, and of which we can hardly discern a trace: the passage of the eagle through the air, the path of a snake across the earth, the traces of a ship across the water, and the path that a man has made inside a young girl.

The existence of the hymen became even less credible when one considered the infinite number of circumstances, excluding any carnal contact, which could produce the same effects as sexual union.

First, there were the dangers arising from the examination itself. Clumsy handling of the genital parts of a woman by ignorant midwives entailed an obvious risk of defloration. Saint Augustine referred to this as early as the third century. In the sixteenth century, Anne Robert criticised in more precise terms those midwives who, 'handling the entire parts of some virgin', destroyed the maidenhead 'out of spite or ignorance'. What virgin could emerge intact from the hands of a midwife who had just probed her 'with a finger, or with a candle or by means of a uterine mirror'?

Midwives were not, however, the only ones to blame. According to Anne Robert's own words, the surgeons were also implicated in these excesses. Armed 'with a male member made of wax', they 'probe the venereal cavity, open it, dilate it, expand and enlarge the parts . . . The maid, even if she be still a virgin, will not emerge other than corrupted and spoiled.' This fact was not lost upon Marie de Corbie, when she declared to her judges that 'if she were found to be other than a virgin maid, this was the work of the physicians and surgeons that did examine her and open her by force when she was visited on the orders of the Court.'

Moreover, what conclusions could possibly be drawn from the examination of a woman who had been subjected over the course of several years of marital cohabitation to an impotent husband's attempts at artificial defloration? 'How,' exclaimed

Guillemeau, 'may you then judge the virginity of a maid who, having lain abed with her husband a thousand times – *et qui eam quoties voluit attretavit jure maritali* [and who, by virtue of his right as a husband has touched her at will], although he has not known her by natural means?'

The supreme argument – and one which afforded a miraculous loophole – of the possibility of manual corruption was more than once cited by deflowered women in legal cases. Marie de Corbie, again, also claimed that it was her husband, Etienne de Bray, who had thus 'opened and dilated her by force . . . Her corruption had indeed been discovered by the surgeons and midwives, she allowed, but she declared that she was deflowered *alio modo quam opere naturali*, adding that her opening and dilation was effected by the defendant *non membre virili, sed alio instrumento: de quo interrogata, respondit se neque ipsum vidisse unquam neque tetigisse* [not with his male member, but with another instrument. Questioned as to the nature of this instrument, she replied that she had never seen it nor touched it].' Later, Marie de Corbie audaciously raised the stakes, by accusing her husband of having carefully premeditated this act of violence with a view to the inevitable trial which would ensue. For whatever practical purposes he had in mind, he used his fingers and 'iron fitments'.

The wife of the Marquis de Langey, Marie de Saint-Simon, defended herself by the same arguments. 'If she no longer appeared to be a maid, it was by the actions of an impotent, and by dint of a passion as furious as it was sterile, which did employ all means to sate itself.' Tallemant de Réaux translated this into more succinct language: 'In the four years that this man has been with her, he has had time and plenty to put her in such condition, be it with his fingers or otherwise, for her to pass as a maid no longer.'

Conversely, any woman brazen enough could, without great difficulty, fit herself with a false virginity, using widely popularised techniques, and thereby sell herself at a higher price to the most fastidious suitor. For the wife keen to be separated from a despised husband, this was the perfect opportunity to pass for a virgin. Jurists were unanimous in denouncing this practice.

From the twelfth century on, Hostiensis, Panorme and other specialists in canon law condemned immodest women who resorted to such means. Surgeons and physicians followed suit. Ambroise Paré compared such 'made-up virgins' to 'whited sepulchres, polished on the outside and filled with corruption and stench inside, as apothecaries' chests are painted without with gold and azure and filled with poison within.'

A singular exception is offered by Dr Venette, whose *Tableau de l'Amour Conjugal* was considered to reflect the most complete bourgeois ethic of the seventeenth century. Yet it contained an obliging inventory of the various prescriptions permitting any fallen woman to pass for the purest slip of a girl. This surprising doctor, however, only overcame his moral scruples after profound meditation and through a sincere burst of philanthropy:

Given the disdain and infamy which may be incurred by an innocent girl who marries when her parts are naturally open, and by another who out of weakness has been led astray by the persuasions of a man that has deceived her, there are sound reasons not to pass over this subject in silence. The peace of families and the husband's peace of mind are almost always re-established by the remedies which it is our intention here to propose.

Elsewhere, Venette comes to the aid of unfortunate women who, in spite of an illicit pregnancy, wish to marry without arousing the suspicions of the spouse. Is it possible, he asks, with a clear conscience to abandon to their sad fate these women whom a passing weakness condemns to eternal debauchery?

To avoid such misfortunes, it was sufficient to submit the vagina to some strange fumigations. Thus, 'the vapour of a little vinegar into which an iron and a red-hot brick have been cast, the astringent decoction of acorn, myrtle, roses of Provins . . . are all remedies which do contract the natural parts of women that are too open.' However, the use of astringents could on occasion prove dangerous. The vapours or liquid entered the womb, the vagina contracted and the genital parts closed up, thus exposing the woman to the painful effects of the corrosive substances.

A century earlier, Ambroise Paré had referred to the pitiful situation of a woman who, despite being pregnant, had the cheek to pass herself off as a 'Saint Catherine' by using astringents. The breach was so well closed that disaster nearly ensued. At birth, the child could not be extracted from his artificial prison, whereupon the genitals had to be cut open to save mother and child just in time.

It was often the mother-in-law who, motivated by pernicious intentions towards her son-in-law, produced an artificial maidenhead. Marie de Corbie used 'sundry restrictives that her mother (a mistress in the art) and a certain other lady, her good friend, had made her to conceal her corruption.'

Some, stronger on realism, brought refinement to such a pitch as to cause a discharge of false blood at the time of the 'first' penetration. 'Since mothers that had immodest daughters,' wrote Anne Robert, 'did slide within the secret parts of the girl a bladder of some fish all smeared with blood, it easily came to pass that the bladder burst and the blood ran forth.'

Paré also criticised those women who 'do insert as deep as the cervix a sponge dipped in the blood of some beast, or fill a bladder in which is contained the choleric humour of sheep,' whereupon 'the poor ninny does believe he has had the cream when he has had only the dregs of the pot.'

For Dr Venette, the same result could be obtained, 'taking a little lamb's blood, heated beforehand, and introducing this into the channel of modesty after fashioning from it two or three small balls.'

Claiming the apparent merit of perfect virginity with impunity was nothing exceptional. Were there not 'wicked and immodest procuresses whose custom it is to sell whores as maids'? 'Today more than ever,' wrote Tagereau, 'there are men and women that will make a girl and virgin out of any woman who has not actually borne a child,' despite which 'the judges of the Church receive these considerations with disbelief and disdain, and do mock when spoken to about these prescriptions.'

Artificial defloration, artificial maidenheads, prescriptions and devices were not sufficient to shock the supporters of the genital examination – for the good reason that they were the very nerve centre of the trial. The preliminary proceedings and the questioning stimulated curiosity, but were never more than the prologue to a deftly executed scenario. The final decision hung fatally upon the inevitable examination report. All the trappings, preparatory show or subsequent commentary on its content, were only gratuitous flourishes whose sole purpose was to entertain the judge, while at the same time giving him his *raison d'être*. The examination was open to endless criticisms, but how could one not see that its abolition would lead to an overall abandonment of legal procedures for the annulment of marriage on the grounds of impotence?

It is easy to understand how the zealots who supported the examination were in a majority.

In fact, there was never a concerted movement for the total abolition of the genital examination. Moreover, its most passionate advocates numbered among their ranks the most relentless defenders of Christian values. At the summit of the ecclesiastical hierarchy, the Court of the Holy Rota in Rome set the example by ordering its continued practice without reservation.

In France, the procurator Lamoignon, who in 1677 was the eulogist of modesty and zealous defender of trial by congress, still saw fit ten years later to approve the initiative of the ecclesiastical judge of Rheims when the latter subjected Pierre Le Gros to proof of erection. And Philippe Hecquet, the pious physician to the nuns of Port-Royal-des-Champs and a relentless pamphleteer on the indecency of midwives, nevertheless brought a devotee's ardour to the task of observing the erections of the Marquis de Gesvres. Furthermore, he declared that, in order to form a sounder opinion of the defendant's condition, 'it would be in order to examine his Lady wife.'

The theologian Le Semelier, an expert in matrimonial matters, was also an avid champion of the examination of women. To call this 'a shameful and scandalous trial' was to forget that 'modesty is but a vain notion when it comes to childbirth.' Modesty was undeniably laudable, 'and the Church that is holy does recognise that the examination is a necessary ill.' But at the end of a subtle argument judiciously combining ambiguity and sophistry, the Church paradoxically emerges with its reputation enhanced, as if sanctified by the act of laying bare the 'shameful parts' of the female members of its flock:

The Church knows how to draw a remedy from sacrilege, and a good of infinite value for glory of Jesus Christ who has raised marriage to the dignity of a sacrament: wise in her conduct, She [the Church] is guided by divine wisdom that has drawn from concupiscence a good as great as the holiness of marriage itself.

Furthermore, this form of trial was probably the only one capable of confounding an impotent husband who perjured himself by affirming under oath that his marriage had been consummated.

The High Court judge Bouhier handled paradox with the same virtuosity, to the point of adapting Saint Ambrose's reservations about undressing nuns to the profit of the supporters of the examination. Ambrose had categorically protested against the attitude of the bishop Syagrius, who wished to determine by such proceedings whether the nun Indicia had really been deflowered. According to Bouhier, however, Ambrose 'pointed out to him that, there being neither proof nor mark against this maid, it was unjust to oblige her to suffer needlessly so mortifying an inspection.' This attitude did not therefore imply any prejudice against the examination as such. This logic was not foolproof, however. Denouncing the incompetence of midwives, Bouhier was forced to recognise by the same token the uncertainty and futility of the examination. 'There would be an extreme danger,' he admits, drawing on the authority of Saint Cyprian, 'of exposing her [the virgin] to the scrutiny of women liable to err, and who by their incompetence could make us suspect a person who is innocent.' Such a fatal and untenable contradiction stripped of any meaning the masterly exposition of an argument culminating in the jurist's declared conviction as to the efficacy of medical inspections.

For the inspection of a woman's genitals was no more shameful than it was inconclusive. This, at least, was one of the tenets of supporters of the examination. There could be no attempt to claim that science was incapable of revealing those shameless women who disguise themselves with a false virginity. All physicians were unanimous that such deceits 'serve only to cover with confusion those women that have used them.' The jurist Gayot de Pitival willingly allowed that there were virginities 'as there are colours for the face, the which are sold over the merchant's counter,' but, he continues:

It is also known that venal virginity does but cover the surface and, regardless of how little one penetrates, it may immediately be seen if it has been purchased for silver. And I would add that there do exist compositions which will make this mask slip.

Constantly referred to and regarded as the supreme authority, the forensic pathologist Zacchia 'dealt with this matter as a doctor, a consultant jurist and an expert on Canon law.' He ruled that virginity can be deduced from six signs. Considered independently of each other, they did not allow the integrity of a woman to be determined, but together they provided certain proof of virginity.

Undeniably, there were fewer sceptics in the eighteenth century than during the previous two centuries. Lost in the mass of supporters of the examination, the theologian Héricourt stressed the inconclusive nature of such a procedure, while the jurist Garat attributed a fortunate purpose to the absence of the hymen – but in vain. The myth of the hymen was a question left unanswered until another era, and the eighteenth century took the most retrograde stand on the issue. Perhaps the abolition of trial by congress served to consolidate the medical examination as the last bastion against the total demise of the impotence trial. This case can be argued, but without it being possible to establish a link of cause and effect between the two phenomena.

In spite of the objections raised by the rare detractors of the examination, and whatever their reasons, it was under the triple protection of the Church, science, and his own conscience that the judge was empowered to order the inspection. However, the unshakable convictions of some commentators can be misleading. In actual fact, inspection of the genitals became a source of controversy, and was always somewhat remote from the passions stirred up by trial by congress. Nor did it elicit the least surprise on the part of contemporaries, since it was generally considered a necessary and normal practice.

The technical and legal conditions of its application, however, posed more delicate problems.

8

In the hands of the experts

The apparent immutability, imperturbable ritual and sang-froid with which the genital examinations were conducted were no more than the attributes of a legal formalism, behind which lurked the most intense passions and often the most impure motivations. A strange question of precedence was the first problem to arise for the judges. Once the examination had been ordered, should the husband or wife be visited first? The seventeenth century did not trouble itself with such subtleties, and Vincent Tagereau declared without beating about the bush that both partners must undergo this trial simultaneously. The eighteenth century proved more finicky and prudish. Inspection of the woman was deemed to compromise modesty, while inspection of the man and trial by erection would on the contrary offend no one. According to the outcome of this first inspection – favourable or otherwise – the couple would be separated or the case dismissed. In either event, the woman would be spared the humiliation of being undressed and having her 'shameful parts' handled. Only when the experts were left in some doubt as to the virile functions of the husband did the ecclesiastical judge resign himself to ordering an examination of the wife. This problem was thus solved with a relative degree of ease. Appointing the experts raised difficulties of another order.

Behind every impotence trial lurked the ominous shadows of midwives, surgeons and physicians, and the judge's sentence was ultimately taken from the findings of these experts.

In the seventeenth century, an impassioned debate arose about the role of midwives in impotence trials. Scholars and

jurists were unanimous: first, by participating in the inspection
of the male genitals they insulted modesty, 'being shameful and
inept, as witness the ridiculous report made by those that
examined De Bray separately, saying that his member was
flaccid and feeble.' Then, like all women, these matrons were
wrong simply by virtue of always thinking themselves right.
'Both judge and public,' lamented the surgeon Guillemeau,
'through what advance information I know not, certainly not
by the operations of reason, do always incline rather to the
report of these women.'

But these inconveniences were minimal in comparison with
the catastrophic consequences which often arose from their
incompetence. This lack of skill was often attributed to their
age. 'Let the judge take care to make his choice with discretion,'
writes Tagereau. 'The midwives must be neither too young nor
too old, since the former lack experience and the latter the sight
and steady hand necessary for such matters. It does therefore
follow that those who use eyeglasses or whose hands tremble
from advancing age shall not be proper to examine women.'

The volatile and quarrelsome character of women was also
naturally incompatible with the gravity of the examination.
'Midwives,' exclaimed Anne Robert, 'do not agree together
and dispute with one another,' so that by the end of an
examination the mystery was usually deeper than at the start.
As for their ignorance, it was manifest. By the end of the
sixteenth century, Joubert was sounding the alarm, saying,
'Matrons may be greatly mistaken, particularly through lack of
instruction in the anatomy of the parts of shame.' According to
Guillemeau, they possessed neither 'reason' nor 'experience',
while the amount of information required to detect male
impotence was quite impressive and depended upon a perfect
anatomical knowledge of the genitals: '. . . of their essence and
perfection in matter, form, temperament, number, magnitude,
appearance, situation and of the connection of one to another:

a matter not to be understood without having had dealings with such parts, not only with the finger but also with the eye.' At the end of the seventeenth century Dr Venette attacked the ignorance of French midwives, recommending that, like Spanish midwives, it would be desirable for them to receive training in anatomy in the schools of medicine.

The terms of this debate became blurred during the eighteenth century. Midwives were admittedly excluded from examinations of males, while surgeons and physicians supervised the examination of females. This controversy, whose twists and turns seem merely to have been the early stirrings of a much more serious conflict, resurfaced again in a different guise and with greater vehemence. If, at a certain point, surgeons and physicians no longer claimed a monopoly over the examination of the genitals, this was because their acquisitive appetites were afforded ample compensation thereafter in the field of obstetrics, an immense new discipline which matched the scale of their ambition – from the end of the seventeenth century, the obstetrician appeared as a formidable rival to the unarmed and 'uneducated' midwife. The former willingly abandoned partial responsibility for inspection of the female, and ceded it to the latter out of charity and in order not to injure the modesty of the female any longer.

Another debate is reflected – though much more diffusely – in certain impotence cases. Here the opponents were physicians and surgeons, each with their respective roles and defined areas of responsibility in the ritual of the genital examination. More generally, this debate emphasised one particular aspect of medical power, illustrated in the seventeenth and eighteenth centuries by the overbearing superiority which physicians displayed towards surgeons. The documents on the Le Gros case are particularly revealing on this point.

Maître Freteau, counsel to Pierre Le Gros, established that the inspection which had been made of his client's genitals ought to be considered 'categorically null'. Contrary to all practice and custom, it had been carried out by two surgeons, in the absence of any representative of the corps of physicians:

It is a certain and observed practice in all physical experiments to summon physicians with surgeons . . . The examination reports can confirm a case of impotence only by supposition and conjecture. Now, supposition and conjecture are operations of a mental and deductive nature (that is to say they are reserved for physicians) and surgeons are entitled only to perform manual operations.

Traditionally, moreover, these manual operations were tainted by prejudice, since 'this part of medicine, which cures only by injury and incisions, was contemplated only with horror.' Physicians, on the other hand, were custodians of

that superior part of medicine which observes the nature of man, and is applied to explore the provinces thereof. The prescriptions which it ordains do distinguish it in kind from the art of the knife and cautery: these are two different professions. It is agreed they do compose a single Faculty, a single Body, but the physician is its head and the surgeon is but its arm.

Aside from its radical version of medical perfection, which is achieved by relegating surgery to the level of butchery, Maître Freteau's discourse also reflects the public conception of the genital examination. The latter was, he claimed, a matter of penetrating

the most secret and hidden parts of the constitution of the accused [Le Gros], there to discover by the force of reasoning and conjecture a principle of weakness [. . .] This great masterwork of detection is reserved for medicine, which is the science of presumptions and conjectures [. . . This is hardly a matter for surgeons, since] it is not permitted them to reason during an anatomical inspection alone, even less is it permitted that they reason on the weakness or inner strength of a living man, during an inspection that is a kind of intellectual anatomy.

Thus the examination of genitals first and foremost resembled an anatomy lesson. The surgeons groped, triturated and dissected, while the physicians reasoned, discussed and conjectured. Ultimately, the Church's sentence depended upon the impulses of these speculative minds.

Against the arguments of Maître Freteau, Maître Bochet was content with defending the strictly objective character of the statement prepared by the surgeons.

They alone are qualified to report on the natural state of a man accused of impotence. Their hands have only to write what their eyes have seen, because it is not upon their judgement that the ecclesiastical judge bases his, it is only on what he has read in their report.

The Church judge himself would be capable of doing the work of the surgeons, but 'the modesty and dignity of his character do not allow him to carry out the inspection.'

Such specious arguments hardly tipped the balance in the surgeons' favour. In effect, the physicians continued to take pride of place. Article 10 of the statutes of the Faculty of Medicine even forbade them to go beyond the limit of manual operations when teaching in the presence of future surgeons.

Moreover, the full weight of the law supported the imperialism of the corps of physicians. By a decree of 5 July 1607, the High Court of Paris forbade surgeons to read a treatise on respiration. The assistant public prosecutor Servin himself declared that 'Science was not for those who had only to do with their hands.' Similar laws forbade them, on pain of heavy sanctions, to undertake any anatomical dissection without the aid of a physician to interpret.

At the beginning of the eighteenth century, the doyen of the Paris medical faculty, Nicolas Andry, decreed that medical students ought also to take courses in surgery. However, this palace revolution stirred up too many prejudices and aroused such hostility that Andry was not re-elected Dean and his reform was repealed.

Under such circumstances it is somewhat surprising that the

High Court of Paris, in the case of Pierre Le Gros, did not invalidate an examination carried out in the absence of physicians. It is true that Le Gros had not been able to 'enter into erection'. It may be assumed that the presence of physicians would have therefore been unnecessary for drawing 'suppositions and conjectures' from so flagrant a case of impotence.

In reality, impotence trials afforded physicians and, in their wake, surgeons and midwives, the opportunity to assert their power. 'In these trials,' exclaimed Le Semelier, 'Faith must be placed in Science, in experience, and in the integrity of the physicians and surgeons.' Theologians and jurists were never at a loss for flattering terms when it came to showering praise upon the medical corps and its decisive interventions in cases of this nature. The complimentary relationship between the medical and judiciary powers is probably not in itself surprising, but the collusion between the ecclesiastical and medical authorities in impotence cases is a fact worthy of attention. In this respect, the style of the experts' reports or of the medical consultations prepared at the request of the Church judge are more than eloquent. Physicians and surgeons never missed the opportunity to make a fine display of their diplomas, naturally, but also paraded unfailingly the references and titles of the clergy by whom their powers were delegated. The medical content of the reports cuts a poor figure beside the unctuous preambles and the procession of illustrious titles.

Nevertheless, a kind of challenge was issued to medical power. This found its earliest expression in the possibility of rejecting experts accused of corruption. In 1640, Estienne Coste declared that, 'the experts being corrupt, they have drawn up so contrived a report that it appears to present some difficulties.' Such accusations were innumerable and often well-founded. They did not, however, undermine either the power or the prestige of experts, but were only one more constituent part of an inexorable routine.

The fundamental criticisms levelled by Vincent Tagereau and Julien Peleus were much more dangerous. Tagereau considered the experts employed by the ecclesiastical courts to be essentially corrupt. They owed their livelihood to the impotence of other men and the supposed virginity of wives. What advantage was there for them in finding men virile or their wives deflowered? Instead, they had powerful motives for falsifying their findings, 'lest they remain useless and without occupation, being only employees of the Church court in these cases, in which they have absolute power.'

Despite these criticisms and accusations, one cannot say that the power of medicine was really challenged by impotence trials. On the contrary, the signatures which appeared at the foot of inspection reports were often those of extremely prestigious doctors.

The recourse to proof by erection was never systematic. Its application was left to the discretion of medical practitioners, who generally only made use of it to disguise their professional incompetence or satisfy their curiosity.

Thus the medical reports were often markedly less obscene when this proof was waived, and some were even couched in terms of great sobriety:

We retired to the chamber of the concierge of the Officiality where we proceeded to examine Nicolas Sene, accused of impotence; having inspected with considerable attention and all possible correctness his natural parts, we discovered these to be normal in number, situation and colour. In consequence of which, we deem that the said M. Sene is possessed of all that is essential in order to consummate the matrimonial act.

Such a degree of discretion was, however, unusual. In the majority of reports we can sense an obvious desire to incriminate, which is most often expressed in complex and awkward terminology. It is as if, at the end of such an elaborate procedure, experts were somewhat reluctant to file a report admitting the virility of the accused, as if this would disappoint or betray the efforts of the learned ecclesiastics. What complicated matters was that excessive simplicity in a report might well be taken for an admission of incompetence. The contents of these reports thus reveal an attitude that was very likely to be detrimental to the person accused.

To increase the impression of certainty in their reports, the experts would try at the outset to extract an admission of impotence from the accused. Where this succeeded, it gave an undeniable stamp of authenticity to the report:

> The aforesaid G.J. today confessed to us that he had never experienced an ejaculation. Signed: Denyau, 7 November 1695.
>
> Having demanded of the aforesaid G.J. if he had been able to achieve carnal knowledge of the petitioner, he told us that no, because he does not have and has never had an ejaculation, having attempted repeatedly, sometimes in the presence of the aforesaid E.P.D. and sometimes alone, without ever having been able to produce any semen. Signed: Thomasseau, 9 November 1695.

In certain cases, manipulation of peripheral observations made it possible to slide imperceptibly from conjecture to certainty:

> We have seen and examined Jean François Doynel, aged 35 years, as he has told us; we did find him to be of a cold and moist humour, and full of bile that has rendered his whole spirit feeble and valetudinarian . . . Signed: Pelletier, Denyau, Courreau, Le Grand, 25 June 1689.
> . . . the aforesaid G.J. is of bad complexion and pale in the face . . .
> G.J. has a poor constitution, and his face is drained of colour . . .
> Henri de Hou throughout his entire body does present the aspect of a doddery old man, and has been thus since he left his mother's womb.

The mention of a deficient complexion augurs badly, for it was considered to be a justification for an unfavourable diagnosis. On occasion it constituted the only evidence. Jean François Doynel was 'feeble and valetudinarian', and this was his only defect, but it was sufficient for the experts to conclude that he was 'incapable of a strong erection when in the company of a woman, ejaculating without intromission; even though all the parts of generation are in order they are without power or vigour.'

Sometimes the accused would appear to be perfectly normal and healthy, as in the case of Henry de Hou. However, from closer inspection the experts decided that 'the genital parts were feeble, malformed, too slack and distended.' By some miracle of eyesight they even noticed that the testicles were full of 'bad bile'. Conclusion: Henry de Hou 'is and will always be irreparably impotent.'

If certain physicians described at length what they had not seen, there were others who went in for extremely realistic descriptions of what they had seen. Pierre Bodard was described as afflicted with a 'foul-smelling indisposition' which the experts accounted for as follows:

We have found upon the scrotum on the left side a suppurating fistulous opening, through which urine does escape involuntarily. (At which point an ulcer has formed.)

The erection is very soft, and there occurs a dissipation of vital spirits which do escape left and right and are not circulated – *in vas debitum* – added to which an irritating indisposition, infected from the involuntary flow of urine which appears through the fistulous ulcer on the scrotum, does hamper the procreative faculties.

Here the diagnosis of impotence rests upon the direct observation of a physical disorder. This would seem to be more rational, and yet in many cases of this kind the experts were not always as strict in their conclusions. Paradoxically, when confronted with an anomaly or a manifest deformity they displayed a greater leniency. A certain L. H. A. had 'a foreskin so tight that the glans may not be uncovered, which must present an obstacle as much to erection as to ejaculation.' But this does not seem to have mattered, for L. H. A. was judged to be potent. A surgical operation would do the rest. Again, one Michel D. P. was unable to consummate the conjugal act because of a phimosis of the foreskin, but the same conclusions were reached and the same verdict of potency.

Ultimately, this attitude of the experts is easily explained. A malformation requiring detailed knowledge could not embarrass them as much as having nothing to report at all, and an optimistic diagnosis did not risk calling into question their abilities. On the contrary, it served as a pretext for a display of erudition, and the message of hope which it emanated could only reinforce the prestigious aura of the medical profession. It was almost better for the accused to present himself to the experts as bearing a slight deformity. Perfection placed them in an awkward situation as well as raising their suspicions.

Everything is ready. The statement appointing the experts has been issued and the inspection comes into legal effect. It takes place most frequently between eight o'clock and eleven o'clock in the morning. There are four experts: two physicians and two surgeons for male inspections and one physician, one surgeon and two midwives for the inspection of females. On the appointed day, they appear before the ecclesiastical court. During the swearing-in, which is presided over by the Church judge, they swear to make a true and objective report. They then proceed to the keeper's room, where the patient is waiting for them and where the surgeons examine and the physicians reason. The report is drafted jointly and sealed. In the event of a difference of opinion, the experts draw up their report separately, presenting as many reports as there are opinions. The document is then forwarded to the judge of the Church and opened in the presence of the experts, who certify it to be true. That is that. It is then up to the judge to make his assessment.

The visit could take a long time. In the case of Claude Hubigneau, it lasted four hours, at the end of which the experts drew up a report whose contents are completely insignificant.

Female inspections took place in different conditions. The

woman was first given a bath of rather peculiar composition in the hope of dissolving any astringents or contrived virginity. The jurist Anne Robert has left a strikingly realistic and audacious account of the examination of a woman. This subject seems to have had a traumatic and lasting fascination for the general public. Several authors refer to it but, out of modesty, usually refrain from quoting. Those who were of this persuasion made a case for condemning the examination as obscene. But the flavour of Anne Robert's style, liberally seasoned with a Rabelaisian spice, cannot fail to impress:

Would you have this spectacle depicted in words? Forgive me, gentle reader whose ears are chaste, if in describing a shameful matter my words do reek of I know not what unchaste and shameful thing. A maid is obliged to lie outstretched to her full length on her back, with her thighs spread to either side so that those parts of shame, that Nature has wished to conceal for the pleasure and contentment of men, are clearly visible. The midwives, matrons all, and the physicians, consider these with much earnest attention, handling and opening them. The presiding judge adopts a grave expression and does hold back his laughter. The matrons in attendance remember old fires, long since cooled. The physicians, according to their age, do recall their first flushes of vigour. The others, seeming busy, do gorge themselves on the vain and futile spectacle. The surgeon, holding an instrument that is fashioned expressly for the purpose, called *the mirror of the womb*, or with a male member made of wax or other matter, explores the entrance to the cavity of Venus, opening, dilating, extending and enlarging the parts. The maid abed does feel her parts itch to such a degree that, even if she be a virgin when examined, she will not leave other than corrupted and spoiled. It would be shameful to speak further of this.

Beyond any doubt however, it was the inspection of a male corpse which was most difficult to justify on moral grounds. The posthumous examination of the Marquis d'Argenton has already been mentioned. A certain degree of scientific curiosity could if necessary be used to disguise the shadier motives, but by no stretch of the imagination could this have been used to justify the post mortem examination of the Count de Coursan.

This was, to say the least, a sinister business. The Comtesse de Coursan had three children baptised under her husband's name. Yet in 1675 she brought a case against her husband alleging that he was impotent. She died soon after, but the case was carried on by her sister, Lady Jacquinot. The Count now followed his wife to the grave. Determined to acquire a separation for the deceased, the zealous sister-in-law immediately set in motion a morbid ballet around his corpse:

Hardly had he passed away when the Lady Jacquinot, in the presence of the civil lieutenant and of the King's procurator of Châtelet, did enter his chamber. Two surgeons that did accompany them inspected his corpse, and after some dissections did draw up their report, declaring that, while all the parts intended for generation were whole and normal in formation, they nevertheless were of the opinion that the Lord of Coursan had only imperfect forces during his life, and that they could achieve the generative act but very imperfectly, the which they did strive to confirm by divers reasonings of their art.

Nor was this all. In his turn, the Count's son demanded

that it be ordered that the body be seen and examined by the physicians of the court, in order that a report be prepared as to the state in which the surgeons of Lady Jacquinot have left it after having cut and hacked at it in divers places. By an order acceding to this request, M. de Mascranni did convey himself to the house, and had a report prepared in his presence concerning the condition in which the corpse was found. The physicians and surgeons of the court, named Rainssant, Turbier and Bienaise, did then declare in their report to have discovered no defect or sign of natural impotence and concluded that the Lord of Coursan could during his life enjoy the practices and actions necessary for generation.

It is as well that the experts did not require proof of erection from the dead Count. Neither the Marquis de Gesvres nor Jacques François Michel were spared on this point.

Proof of erection was the main aim of the genital examination of men. Here, the sin of Onan was raised to the level of an institution of canon law. This strange paradox can only be explained and justified by the confusion of experts when confronted by the impotence of perfectly formed men. Eighteenth-century commentators traditionally traced the 'proof of erection', of 'natural movement' or of 'elastic tension' back to the twelfth century. Hostiensis, the Cardinal of Suze, did indeed specify that the judge must satisfy himself regarding the motor faculties of the accused, since lack of erection constituted proof of impotence. In fact, it is not certain that proof of erection had been required since that time, and the interpretation of the jurists of the classical period reflected above all their own concern to invest this trial with the legitimacy conferred by history. In the last analysis, everything depended upon the meaning given to the verb *inquirere*. Was it necessary for the judge to 'satisfy himself' by demanding proof of erection? Could he not determine this in a more subtle manner during the cross-examination, the preliminary enquiry or by recourse to the *septima manus*?

Certainly the proof of erection had been a well established procedure since the late sixteenth century, when Antoine Hotman and Vincent Tagereau discussed it in detailed terms.

It cannot be said that this trial caused any great indignation. Tagereau, while shocked by trial by congress, was content to note that the experts might require the accused 'to endeavour to stand erect, in which task he may be aided by legitimate means which the art of medicine teaches.'

A century later, Le Semelier recognised that

there is great indecency in this examination – *quia vir provocatur ad libidinem* [because the man is subjected to libidinous provocation] – whence it follows that the ecclesiastical judge, who should be attached to the purity and morality of the Gospel, must order it only after prudently examining whether the parties are acting and complaining with sound reason.

And from Boucher d'Argis came the astonishing caution: 'There can be no doubt that proof of natural movement may be ordered, but the experts and midwives must take great care not to exceed their mission.' A heavy hint indeed.

Some went even further. At the end of the seventeenth century, the forensic pathologist Zacchia considered that erection was not even absolute proof of virility. 'Some,' he wrote, 'in spite of the most flattering appearances, are nevertheless incapable of effecting penetration and ejaculation into the appropriate orifice.'

The intransigent Bouhier further specified that, 'while the elastic faculty in a man is the principal sign of virility, it is nevertheless not of itself sufficient – *nisi coire vere possit* [unless the man can actually achieve coitus].' From this point to ordering a 'trial by ejaculation' was only a short step which certain experts may well have taken.

When the accused was called upon to exhibit his virile talents, he was granted a number of 'privileges': the choice of the time and place for the trial, for example. In the event of failure, he was offered further chances to prove himself. The experts were very 'tolerant' on this matter. The Marquis de Gesvres and Jacques François Michel were set to work time after time. One attempt followed another: four, five, six . . . and all in vain. Occasionally the house of the accused was the setting for these sad capers. The unfortunate man lay on his bed, shrinking underneath the blankets. The experts waited at hand. The patient aroused himself, was uncovered, examined, patted, measured and the report drawn up. On occasion, the fantastic was combined with the sinister.

A villager from the Rheims region, Pierre Le Gros, was the unfortunate spouse of Martine Le Brun who, after two years of living with her husband, sought to end the marriage on the grounds of non-consummation. The case came up on appeal before the High Court of Paris in 1687. First he was accused of having only one testicle and no beard. Second, and most important, he was considered incapable of a state of erection. Understandably so, since he had been in the very act of attempting to shake off his torpor, in the presence of two surgeons, when his wife's father, her counsel and two strange surgeons had burst into his home and insulted him:

It was attempted [said Le Gros' lawyer] to effect this examination in a rush . . . Thus, how could the appellant, agitated by choler, surprised by the great haste, held back by modesty, trembling in the fear of a poor outcome, and amidst all this pressed by his own impatience, not succumb, since all the spirit and the heat of manhood could barely suffice to defy the divers movements of so many contrary passions.

The conviction on appeal of Pierre le Gros was a fact of capital importance. For it took place on the strength of the conclusions of the assistant public prosecutor, Lamoignon, who, ten years earlier, had supported the abolition of congress trials. It proved that this austere champion of modesty, by giving his backing to the proof of erection, intended to demonstrate that there was nothing in common between the two procedures.

Thirteen years later, Florent Cahu experienced a similar situation. His wife, Françoise Messand, dragged him before the ecclesiastical court of Blois. On 16 September 1700, the experts ruled him to be of normal physical formation. This, however, was by no means sufficient. 'Thus, to learn whether he had any internal defect, all requested unanimously that he should present an erection in their presence, to judge in this manner any defect of the inner parts.' The result was so pitiful that the experts attributed it to fear. They left him alone for a considerable time. On their return, they found Cahu in the same state. All his efforts, he declared ingenuously, had been fruitless. The experts magnanimously extended the period until the next day. 'They promised to come to where he lay abed, so that with a delay he might more easily come to heat and content them in this matter . . . but the following morning he confessed a second time to having no erection, still less ejaculation.'

The Le Gros and Cahu cases afford a foretaste of a reality which teetered into the fantastic when De Gesvres and Jacques François Michel faced their experts.

In the De Gesvres case, legal procedure turned into dementia. It is difficult to imagine today the passions and the gravity of the problems raised by the hypothetical erections of the Marquis de Gesvres. On 3 June 1709, Joachim Bernard Poitier, the Marquis de Gesvres, married at the age of nineteen Marie Magdeleine Emilie Mascranni. Three years later, the latter filed a suit with the ecclesiastical court of Paris on the grounds of her husband's impotence. The cross-examination took place on 20 April 1712 and, on 24 May, the accused underwent the first of a long series of physical examinations. The experts signed two separate but not contradictory reports:

> We saw and closely examined the Marquis de Gesvres and found his external parts adapted to fructification were proper as to their appearance, bulk and size; but, as these conditions do not suffice to judge as to the consummation or otherwise of a marriage, erection and ejaculation being required, and as these were not revealed to us, we may not absolutely decide whether he be in condition to satisfy the duties of marriage.
>
> Drawn up in Paris, this twenty third day of May, 1712, Signed: Gayant and Marechal.

Hecquet and Chevalier came to identical conclusions but added that 'it would be appropriate to examine the person of Madame Mascranni.' After his first inspection, therefore, doubts were left hanging over the Marquis's manly capacities, and the matter was open to the most diverse interpretations. The controversy drew in the opposing figures of the counsel for the Marquis, Maître Chevalier, and the Marquise's lawyer, Maître Begon.

'He has the form, therefore he has the movement,' cried the former.

'If the Popes had reasoned thus, we would surely have no term "De Frigidis et Maleficiatis",' the other replied drily.

'The unfortunate Marquis has been given notice to exhibit his manly vigour in the presence of four gentlemen capable of extinguishing the most ardent of fires.'

'Perhaps so. But these experts possess the art of submitting their patient to all manner of prickings and spurs . . . They have secrets to excite movement, tinglings to prick sensitivity. Such excitations are by no means wrong when employed only to inform the Church.'

'What are these alleged secrets reserved for those of the art? It might be said that they are the notions of an orator who does let his imagination roam. But what are these alleged permitted excitations? It might be said that they are blasphemies . . .'

On 3 April 1713, the second examination took place, and there was still no sign of an erection. The report does, however, allow with a degree of cynicism 'that there are men for whom the presence of other men is an obstacle to erection', which might, at a pinch, pass for mitigating circumstances. Maître Begon was outraged by this suggestion: would the physicians and surgeons wish perchance 'to induce us to entrust the inspection of M. de Gesvres to persons of the other sex?' In spite of this outburst, the outcome of the second trial left him entirely satisfied. 'Not only,' he concluded, 'is the form insufficient, but not even the notion of ardour or movement signifies when such movement is entirely bereft of firmness and hardness.'

The experts expressed the wish 'that M. le Marquis be allowed to have his Er . . . in our presence, at another time and in another place more favourable to him.'

These were the conditions in which the ruling of 23 August 1713 took place. The accused received 'permission to be visited and examined at a time and in such suitable quarters as he shall indicate to the experts.'

Thus, on the twenty-first of the same month, early in the morning, the physicians Daval and Littre and the clerk of the court Ysabeau arrived at the Hotel de Tresme in the Rue Neuve-Saint-Augustin, where the Marquis lived, and arranged an obscene piece of theatre.

'We did find him in a state of erection upon our arrival,' states a first report, 'but he did not have sufficient attributes to consummate a marriage.' A second report was more detailed:

We found him abed, awake already and awaiting us impatiently. Two surgeons that were in the ante-chamber admitted us, and we examined the virile member on three different occasions, at around one half hour's interval each from each, as invited by one of the afore-mentioned surgeons who were coming and going between the chamber of the Marquis and the antechamber to which we were conducted after each examination. On every occasion we did indeed observe that the part to be Er . . . , that is to say distended and hard; but the tension, hardness and duration in this condition did not appear to us as sufficient for the act of generation.

The Marquis's virility seems to have been a decidedly ephemeral phenomenon, and the experts were once again perplexed. A fourth visit was required. Two days later they returned to work, but on this Monday, August 23, an unforeseen circumstance awaited them. Having waited impatiently for three quarters of an hour, they were informed that 'the Marquis was not in a condition to be examined, since he had the stomach aches and even felt prone to vomit, through having supped to excess on the previous evening.' And the Marquis having 'supped to excess' on the previous evening, the experts left without being able to satisfy their thirsts.

Maître Chevalier's somewhat embarrassed explanation ran like this: 'The Marquis did not know on the Sunday evening that he was to be examined on the Monday morning. The conveyance of experts was arranged by his family, unbeknownst to him, for fear that the idea of the examination might freeze his imagination during the night and, finally, since he was not expecting the examination, he abandoned himself to his appetite in the course of the evening.'

A specious argument, retorted Maître Begon. The Marquis had woken at eight o'clock, and imposed a wait of three-quarters of an hour upon the experts, and only then did he become aware of his bad indigestion . . .

Weeks passed, and then months. Maître Begon became impatient. 'Make your simulacra move! Move them, Marquis!' he cried out in open court. In February 1714, 'having reflected for six months,' the Marquis decided finally that he was ready to comply with the ruling of 2 August. The lawyer of his wife, the Marquise, recalled that this involved 'entering into the state demanded by the report of the 3rd of April . . . and in accordance with this principle, the Marquis de Gesvres was required to present to the experts no mean movement but one which was firm and lasting.'

In fact, last minute upsets delayed the final trial: on 2 March, an erysipelas, on 7 March an outbreak of green scabies, in April a sore, in July nausea, and so on. 'What itch, what scabies, Monsieur le Marquis?' enquired Maître Begon ironically. 'Perchance a scabies wearing the livery of the Spanish fly [aphrodisiac] that you were obliged to take?' When the Marquis decided to face the experts, he was again found to be in a state of the deepest lethargy. Maître Begon was exultant: 'The experts who visited him in 1714 have found him moulded on the model they drew in 1713.' They did observe something stirring, but it was only

a movement lacking in the required qualities, insufficient in its tension, in its hardness, in its duration . . . without counting the great and violent reasons for presuming that this very movement was no more

than an artificial imitation of nature . . . all concurred in rejecting as
coin of the poorest alloy this manner of movement which M. de
Gesvres did present.

'Let other experts examine my client,' cried out Maître
Chevalier. 'Dupre and Sarramia, for example.'

'Out of the question,' interjected Begon. 'These you mention
are ordinary surgeons of the house, all persons in the livery of
the Hotel de Tresmes, capable of falsifying and so to speak
adulterating the human body so as to delude justice in a matter
of the sacrament of marriage.'

The response to this was extraordinary.

'My erection,' declared the Marquis, 'is for the eyes of Dupre
and Sarramia alone, but as for you, critical and superstitious
experts, just looking at you makes me wilt. After all, how can
you expect to see that which your very presence puts to rout?
Content yourselves, therefore, with what you do see, and by
that token imagine what you do not see.'

For three long years this lamentable case dragged on amidst
violent outbursts until, weary of the war, the Marquise withdrew the case against her husband in 1717, although not before
receiving substantial damages. She died the same year, at the
age of twenty-five, undermined, it was said, by the profound
chagrin occasioned by this sad affair. 'The Marquise de Gesvres, wife of the Marquis de Gesvres, has died. It was she that
attempted the famous impotence trial on which two extremely
curious volumes have been compiled,' wrote Mathieu Marais
in his *Journal* for 9 July 1717.

Some years later, another bravura piece was played out. Jacques François Michel, a good bourgeois draper of Amiens, was
arraigned before the ecclesiastical court of Beauvais at the
request of Suzanne de Machy, his dissatisfied wife. The trial
began in 1735 and ended in 1740.

Our man defended himself as best he could, but the final

word rested with the experts who, over a period of five years, gave free rein to their fantasies. From seven examinations and some fifteen reports, nothing certain emerged. More than ten physicians and surgeons succeeded each other at the bedside of François Michel, including eminent 'specialists' in sexual problems: Andry, Winslow and Dionis. Some decided to employ radical means. They installed themselves permanently in the house of the accused in the hope of surprising, scrutinising and analysing the least signs of an erection. The doctors Croissant de Garengeot and Col de Vilars spent whole nights in the small apartment which the accused rented in Paris and where the appeal case was heard.

The first report contained nothing decisive. The doctors Fontaine and Russel reported 'sufficient form' but as a consolation, gave themselves wholeheartedly to a tangle of peripheral observations:

We did find the bags, or scrotum, more distended and more spacious than is correct, all the cutaneous glands of the said scrotum being hardened and exceeding the size of a grain of millet; the interior of the membranes common to the testicles and the sperm ducts, principally on the left side, presented the consistency of cotton to the touch . . . We did perceive on the anus divers rather swollen haemorrhoids, and the extremity of the internal membrane of the rectum turned outwards, thus making a large, inflamed and very irritated fold . . .

'In the very slight doubt in which we find ourselves,' the experts added pleasantly, 'we did enquire of M. Michel if he had erections, whereupon he replied he did have one almost every day.'

The following day, another inspection:

We found M. Michel abed, did inspect and examine him, and at first perceived his penis to be a little larger and raised than on the previous occasion, the which he termed a weak erection and which we would esteem to be none at all.

Further peripheral matters were mentioned: 'We found the bags less spacious than on the occasion of the first examination ... the anus was in its natural state ...'

Alongside these anatomical observations, a legal quarrel was developing. In the opinion of Jacques François Michel's lawyer, Messrs. Simon, Fontaine and Russel had been chosen inadvisedly by Suzanne de Machy. They were 'young, incompetent and partial'. Their reports reeked of 'ignorance, temerity and prevarication'. For François Michel could indeed show an erect penis, although admittedly a limited one. But the unfortunate man,

believing he could trust in the whims of nature, did promise to show them on the following morning the sign which they awaited. He did not deceive them. It is true that he did not show it to them in its highest degree, but only in its decline. These were the embers of a fire which had been lit and gone out. M. Michel, who, when the experts presented themselves at the street door, was in a state of the most accomplished erection ... having, however, no servant at home to open for them, he was obliged to leave his bed, to descend from the room and to cross a courtyard in his shirt and breeches to admit the experts ... At the end of the month of August, the mornings do begin to be chill. The disturbance caused by the presence of four experts must be added to this consideration ... The experts recognised this, and did leave M. Michel the space of some minutes to return to his bed and recover a little his spirits; but Nature did not see fit to remount to that zenith which it had reached earlier ...

Such, according to Maître Simon, were the circumstances deliberately omitted in the experts' report. But this unfairness was relatively innocuous compared to the audacity of the physicians Croissant de Garengeot and Col de Vilars who, 'following on the above events, dared to conduct their examination, or rather their banditry, with a patent insincerity and lack of faith.'

And indeed, one morning in April, these two gentlemen did appear at the 'Rue Champfleury, at the house of M. Gautier, renter of furnished rooms, at the apartment occupied by M. Jacques François Michel, good bourgeois and merchant of Beauvais.'

Their investigations began with a measuring session:

> We found M. Michel abed and started by inspecting his natural parts in their relaxed state, the better to judge the difference in the erections that he might present.

These experts then proceeded to install themselves in the adjacent vestibule and await further developments. Time passed. A day, a night, a second day, a second night. Then, suddenly . . .

> . . . at a quarter to three we lent our ears to a sort of agitation and movement that M. Michel was making, and we did hear his breathing to be troubled, tight and short. Whereupon he called out to us and we did instantly go to his bed with a lit candle. We observed that he used only his left hand to raise the cover and, assisting him, we saw that his right hand, which he promptly withdrew, was covering his pubis . . . We found his member swollen in its cavernous tissue . . . Touching this swelling, we felt it to be flabby . . . In short this swelling of the cavernous body did endure barely the space of half a minute and, far from lasting longer upon being handled, as is the case with the true erection, it immediately faded away.

Monsieur Simon here leapt at his opportunity:

> What penis, he exclaimed, however swollen it might be, when handled and examined by Garengeot (since M. Col de Vilars was content to hold the candle all the time) would not wilt on the very spot? Did this oracle from Bourges flatter himself that he was of sufficiently comely appearance and had a sufficiently enlivening hand to stroke the imagination of a man of modesty?

During the entire period of his torture, the patient could manage no better. He struggled like the devil to give his examiners the least pitiful impression of him possible. Resorting to heavy understatement, the physicians attempted to draw a case for a 'guilty' verdict from this manifest impairment.

We observed at the same time that M. Michel was out of breath, his respiration being troubled, his eyes and face red, with large drops of sweat running down the latter. Seeming himself to be surprised by this state, he told us that he had just awoken, although we had perceived his agitation and movements for a quarter of an hour before he summoned us.

On 27 April 1739, a further surprise lay in wait for Jacques François Michel. Experts again appeared at his door to proceed with the examination ordered by a ruling of 14 March 'which,' they said with cynicism, 'did admit M. Michel to trial by erection.' The watch was mounted. At three in the morning, the accused finally became erect. But, said the experts, can one speak of erection when 'at the time, he had the benefit of the moment when a bladder full of urine does ordinarily cause a species of erection?' A quarter of an hour later, Jacques François Michel again called the experts to his bedside. Alas! 'He uncovered himself only with the left hand while the fingers of the right pressed the root of the penis . . .'

On balance: Was the erection weak? It was not to be relied upon. Was it real? It was assigned a doubtful cause – a full bladder, the right hand under the covers . . . in addition to which it had the great misfortune to fade away when first touched by the physician.

Physical suffering was added to moral suffering when the experts decided to introduce a stylet into the urethra of the unfortunate victim, 'to judge the force of the action of the generative parts.'

During the fifth examination, the doctors Andry and Mongin became outraged by 'this rash means, which could only expose him to injury and suffering.' For their part, they preferred the urine test:

It is sufficient, soundly to gauge the facility with which the spermatic humour may pass through the channel of the urethra, to have him urinate, as we advised M. Michel to do, the which he did in our presence at full stream and to a great distance.

In spite of all these misadventures and the humiliating uncertainties by which Jacques François Michel was implicated, four of the reports were in his favour. Severity nevertheless won the day, and the judges, relying on the authority of the most pessimistic reports, found in favour of Suzanne de Machy. Jacques François Michel was declared impotent and, by a decision of the Great Chamber dated 11 August 1740, there was found to have been 'no injustice in the verdict of the ecclesiastical court of Beauvais,' as a result of which the marriage was declared null and void, and the accused ordered to pay a fine.

It may easily be imagined that, in such circumstances, uncertainties plagued the progress and the resolution of many cases. It was in order to resolve these uncertainties that the astonishing institution of trial by congress was introduced into France in the mid-sixteenth century.

9

Trial by congress

From about 1550 onwards, trial by congress dominated the proceedings of the ecclesiastical courts. The power of this physical test of sexual potency to arouse violently strong emotions in the public meant that the impotence trial itself came to occupy a position of central importance. At the same time it provoked a crisis in which the institution of the trial as a whole was soon to become embroiled. Congress bewitched and traumatised the public imagination. The judges, though fascinated by it, deplored its obscene character, without however being able to bring themselves to abolish it. The accused, who were more than likely to fail this ordeal, loudly demanded their right to undergo it. De Bray, De Langey and many others precipitated themselves towards it like so many moths around the flame.

In this trial, the real and the unreal were mingled in the strangest manner, for the carnal act consummated in the presence of witnesses constituted, of course, irrefutable evidence of virility, yet this act did not number among those normally carried out in public by order of a judge. Here were two mutually exclusive premises which served to nourish the extraordinary controversy which evolved around the trial by congress. Everyone demanded its abolition on the grounds of immorality, but nobody really took it upon themselves to prohibit it. In the face of storms and tempests, the solitary 'monster' stood its ground. Pursuing a comfortable existence in the midst of the upheavals which surrounded it, the trial by congress succumbed only in 1677, its final death-blow meted out by the assistant public prosecutor, Lamoignon. But by a further paradox, it survived in a kind of after-life until the beginning of the nineteenth century, its memory faithfully preserved in a multitude of fascinated and nostalgic descriptions which wistfully denounced its obscene character.

The inexhaustible propensity for paradox which characterised the institution of trial by congress was embedded in the very etymology of the term. 'Congress: an action in which two beings draw together by matching each other in single combat.' In Latin, *congressus* signifies an encounter, an attack, but also sexual commerce. In old French, 'le congrès' referred primarily to the act of love. Ambroise Paré spoke of 'the irresistible desire for congress' which animates both men and women. To phrase this differently, however, the two protagonists engage in a 'virile combat', in which the 'warrior' employs his 'lance' to penetrate the lair of procreation.

Germanic law and the judgement of God were never far away. From amorous combat to carnal ordeal was a short step, and the notion of a duel enacted before the eyes of the law imposed itself early on. 'The shamelessness and corruptions of the age,' wrote Anne Robert, 'desire and ordain that a wife be permitted to provoke her husband into combat. This combat is termed congress . . . The royal ordinances do forbid the practice of duelling between noblemen, yet there exists no law forbidding duels and combats between those soldiers that do engage under the flag of Venus.'

'With regard to Congress,' remarked Sébastien Roulliard, 'we may say that duelling is clearly forbidden by the edicts, but not that kind which does occur between man and wife.'

During the seventeenth and eighteenth centuries, the term retained its belligerent overtones. Thus in the actual words of the jurists, 'the Lord and Lady de Langeais were left to fight it out, in the course of that congress which did bring them into conflict before the eyes of the justice.' But more legalistic definitions began to supplant the metaphorical usages:

Congress: the venereal act between a man and a woman, as ordered by a decision of the court.

Congress: the trial of potency or impotency of married couples, as ordained by the law in times past, and which took place in the presence of surgeons and matrons on the occasions when it involved the annulment of a marriage on the grounds of impotency.

The origins and antiquity of congress are disputed. The Greek poet Lucian was frequently cited as a source, who in 'The Eunuch' referred to the controversy which had sprung up in a literary circle concerning a certain Bagoas. Was it proper to admit the latter to the ranks of philosophy professors despite his beardless face and high-pitched voice? Some proposed that, in order to decide upon his virility with full knowledge of the facts, he should be exposed publicly to the charms of a courtesan. But seventeenth-century jurists were unanimously agreed on one point: that this harmless joke, despite sharing vague similarities with congress, could be no substitute for a proper legal antecedent. Dr Venette was the only one to support the view of a historical origin for congress. He claimed that the trial was practised in Roman law up until the reign of Justinian, who abolished it. But according to Bayle's *Dictionnaire*, this error arose from 'some transposition of ideas', by which Venette confused the examination sanctioning puberty, which was indeed abolished under the instigation of Justinian, with trial by congress.

In the last analysis, psychology was preferred to history, and commentators were more interested in castigating judges and couples alike. 'There is every indication,' wrote Antoine Hotman, 'that congress was introduced not so much by the judges, as by appointment to the couples themselves, given that they do offer themselves up to it so willingly.' Tagereau was more accurate when he suggested that congress owed its existence to 'some shameless fellow who, being prosecuted by the law and boasting that he could make apparent his potency, probably demanded such a trial . . . the which may well have been granted him in order to discourage the women from undertaking impotence suits in the first place.'

A century and a half later, the compilers of the *Journal du Palais* voiced a similar hypothesis. The 'temerity of some young man' was considered in all probability to underlie the institution of congress. But above all it was the moral responsibility of judges which was at issue in these controversies, because their turn of mind 'is always seeking new means to discover the truth of obscure matters.' Above all, the institution of congress was thought to flourish thanks to its pernicious exploitation by women, 'who know, one and all,' said Hotman, 'that it is an unfailing means for them to win their cases.' This argument was taken up in chorus by Tagereau and Venette. For the latter, who was an incorrigible misogynist, congress was 'merely a pretext for divorce, and an invention of the lasciviousness of womankind. It is they themselves who planted in the minds of judges the inspiration for a trial which is as obscure as it is dishonest.'

The simplest explanation is that congress was probably instituted by judges and physicians who were perplexed by the phenomenon of perfectly formed but impotent men. This invention, despite its scabrous and inquisitorial character, seemed to afford an incontrovertible means of proof. More generally, it was of course a manifestation of the determined and morbid will to knowledge, at whatever price, which typified the age.

A primitive version of trial by congress seems to have been practised for the first time in Spain during the fifteenth century. In this connection, the canonist Sanchez described the confusion of Spanish judges and experts when confronted by the dilemma of a widow, clearly no longer a virgin, and her second husband who was accused of impotence but was physiologically normal. At the demand of his wife, he was forced to allow matrons into the conjugal bedchamber as witnesses. By what route this practice came to be introduced into France and then flourish during the sixteenth and seventeenth centuries remains a mystery.

The fact that it was a very recent phenomenon was undisputed. Hotman and Tagereau dated the first case of trial by congress to around the mid-sixteenth century. Bouhier, defying the unanimous opinion of other commentators, assigned to it a more respectable age. But one must take into account that this mid-eighteenth century champion of congress was preoccupied, in a belated and nostalgic manner, with according the institution its patent of nobility.

The same sentiment motivated Bouhier when it came to proving how widespread this practice was. According to him, it was common in Italy, England and the Low Countries. For the latter two countries, Bouhier's argument rested upon slender grounds. But it is possible that some form of trial by congress was intermittently practised in Spain, and more systematically in Italy. The testimony of Petrus de Ancharano rests upon a curious account of a member of the ecclesiastical court of Venice who incarcerated a man and a prostitute in the same room. On the basis of the latter's version of what occurred, the marriage of this unfortunate man was annulled. But the collected verdicts of the Holy Rota, the ecclesiastical court in Rome, which Zacchia described in detail, bear far more eloquent testimony to the historical antecedents of congress. They include the case of a husband presumed impotent who, by order of the examining physicians, was forced to undress and go naked to bed with his wife (*solus cum sola, nudus cum nuda in communi lecto*). The couple were left alone and, at the end of this trial, which lasted two hours, the conjugal act was deemed not to have been performed. It would even appear that congress, which was abolished in France in 1677, survived for a longer period in Italy, since Maître Begon refers to 'this infamous trial which has in our day been sent back beyond the Alps, whence it came.'

But whatever its actual geographical extent, congress remained a peculiarly and specifically French institution, and this is precisely how it was regarded by contemporaries. 'By what misfortune,' exclaimed the correspondent of the *Journal du Palais*, 'does it [congress] come to be accepted in France alone? How can a nation that is distinguished from all others by its genuine honesty, harbour among the holy and judicious laws which do govern it, a custom so contrary to morals and even to truth itself?'

It is difficult, if not impossible, to assess the frequency with which trials by congress took place. The sources are far too incomplete and, unlike the medical visit, congress was entirely unsystematic in its workings. The common consensus of the time ascribed to it an increasing regularity. According to Venette, 'there are many more dissolutions of marriage these last hundred years or so, since congress came into existence, than were to be seen hitherto.' 'The annals of our jurisprudence,' observed Gayot de Pitival, 'do enshrine a host of memorials attesting that this indecent trial was ordained and confirmed by a multitude of decrees.' Etienne Pasquier actually furnished the curiosity of the public with an imposing list of the great victims of congress: 'It is through congress that were judged the cases of the Lord Hames, the Lord Senarpon; those of Turpin, Lord of Assigny, of Erasme de la Tranchée, of Baron de Courcy . . .'

This impression must nevertheless be tempered by the more sober reality. It is probably not surprising that the sensational character of trial by congress should have left in its wake such vivid recollections. But it is precisely this astonishing literary efflorescence around a relatively limited number of cases which

prompts us to be cautious. For the Quellenecs, the De Brays
and the De Langeys recur again and again in the accounts of all
the commentators. Ecclesiastical judges could not abuse the
institution of congress without bringing down upon themselves the hypocritical rage of their puritanical courts. The
opprobrium which the High Court of Paris heaped upon the
ecclesiastical court of Coutances, which had ordered trial by
congress for a man of over seventy years old, was hardly
encouraging.

In spite of this, there must have lurked in the depths of every
ecclesiastical court the sweet hope that, one day, it might be
able to treat itself to the luxury of a trial by congress. Even if the
victim were an old man, the possibility of ordering such an
ordeal would be exciting enough. How otherwise can we
explain the endurance, over a period of centuries, of an obscene
and notoriously inefficient institution? Concerning this luxury,
one ecclesiastical judge, a friend of Ménage, confessed to having
savoured it once in his career:

A judge of the time of M. de Condi, whose name I can no longer recall,
once told me that during the forty years that he exercised his responsi-
bilities, he had ordered a congress on but one occasion. The man was a
joiner. In the midst of the trial, as he was performing his duties in
exemplary fashion, his wife said to him: why did you never do thus
when we were at home, and there would have been no need for us to
come here?

The conduct of these trials brought the law's extravagance in
such matters to a fever pitch. And, as if trial by congress were
not already sufficiently bizarre, it was to become further
embroiled in a ritual which can hardly be said to have lacked
imagination.

Moreover, the institution of congress seems to have been
firmly rooted in custom, since, outside judicial trials, the notion
of a private or familial trial was not considered to be in any way
shocking or extraordinary. The Marquis de Langey actually

proposed it to his wife's family, and Henri Fermier submitted to it in 1662, without success, for 'having made congress in the presence of divers relatives,' he was forced to admit to being impotent. Twenty-three years after the official abolition of trial by congress in 1677, we find Claude Hubigneau agreeing to demonstrate his virility in front of his parents-in-law, at the injunction of his wife's mother, who 'was desirous of witnessing the conjugal act that he would perform in her presence.'

Yet congress could be legally enforced only through the decision of a judge, in which case a refusal to perform implied automatic guilt. Trials could vary in length from a couple of hours to several days. Thus the jurist Chenu praised the thoroughness of the ecclesiastical judge of Albi, who ordered one couple to pass three consecutive nights in the presence of matrons. In the majority of cases the trial would take place on neutral ground, in a rented room for example. Sometimes relatives and friends would escort the two partners to the appointed place and wait in an adjoining room together with the justice delegates.

The experts who were in attendance on these occasions would insist upon a long rigmarole of precautions to exclude the possibility of fraud. Tagereau, who left a particularly faithful account of trial by congress, explains the procedure as follows:

Both parties are examined all naked, from the crown of the head to the soles of the feet and in all parts of their bodies – *etiam in podice* – to find if there be any thing upon their person as might assist or harm the congress.

[To prevent the use of astringents] the woman is put in a shallow bath where she does remain some period of time.

[Next is examined] the state of the privy parts, by such means to establish the difference betwixt their extent of expansion and distention before and after the congress, and if intromission hath occurred or no.

After this the trial proper could commence.

This being done, the man and wife do betake them to bed in broad day, and the experts that are present do either remain in the bedchamber or retire away (if the parties or one of the parties require this) to some garderobe or gallery close by, the door remaining however at jar, and as for the matrons they do stay around the bed. And the curtains of which then being drawn, it is the duty of the man to set to making proof of his potency, whence often there arise nonsensical disputes and altercations, the husband complaining that his partner will not permit him to perform and does hinder intromission, his wife the while denying the charge and claiming that he would put his finger therein and dilate and open her by such means alone . . .

[Tagereau reckons that it would take] a marvellous determined man and even brutish not to turn flaccid, assuming him to be already in a state of excitation. And if nonobstant such indignities and obstacles he carry on even unto intromission, this were impossible unless the legs and arms of his partner were to be held down . . .

At the last, the parties having passed some time abed, like one hour or two, the experts being called or, weary of waiting, do of their own accord approach and open the curtains, to discover what hath taken place between the couple. The woman is examined close up, to discover if she be more dilated than on the last inspection before her retiring to bed, and whether intromission has occurred (and if there be an emission, and where, and of what nature). This is conducted without the use of candles or those spectacles worn by people advanced in age, though not without exceedingly profane and shameful inspection and argumentation. And they do make up their reports which they deliver to the judge that is in the same house, installed in a separate room or chamber together with the prosecutors and patricians of the ecclesiastic courts that do await the end and issue of the act, which report always disadvantages the man, unless he hath achieved intromission.

In accordance with the same scenario, De Bray was subjected to three trials in succession. According to his lawyer, the situation was made even more unbearable by the flagrantly indelicate behaviour of his wife, the youthful Mademoiselle de Corbie. The second trial, at which the experts were present, took place under particularly dramatic circumstances:

The man De Bray was examined from the soles of his feet to the crown of his head, including all the concavities and secret parts of his body, this being done much less to determine if he had anything hid about his person that might assist him in performing the said act of congress, than to vex him in order that he might leave the field.

Moreover, Mademoiselle de Corbie provoked an absurd argument concerning 'the bonnets that they would wear upon their heads, so that some of these had to be sent out for from the Petit Pont.' Meanwhile, the time allotted for De Bray to accomplish his task was running out, his chances of success were diminishing, and his virile ardour was flagging. To add insult to injury 'the plaintiff [his wife] did give vent to an infinity of scandalous and injurious expressions for to anger him and distract him from his undertaking.' De Bray's nerves had already been shattered by the postponement of several previous trials at the insistence of his shrewish wife, who claimed either to be 'having her months' or that 'the sheets of the bed were poisoned . . .' In the end, however, De Bray seemed to triumph over all the odds: 'the doctors and matrons do all report having seen and touched his member, that it was big, stiff, red and long, and that it was in place and in good order to perform the said congress.' And yet he subsequently lost the case, on the grounds that he had superfluously scattered a 'too aqueous and serous' seed around the edges of the appropriate orifice.

With the trial of René de Cordouan, the Marquis de Langey, the law abandoned the last vestiges of restraint. By now the institution of congress was clearly at its apogee, although the end was not far away. For the unexpected sequels to the De Langey trial were to provoke a violent reaction on the part of the state prosecutor against the procedure as a whole.

Here we may recall the frenzied uproar which surrounded the De Langey affair. Admittedly the behaviour of the Marquis was not exactly calculated to calm things down. In his wounded pride he omitted no opportunity to draw attention to himself by ill-timed and extravagant gestures. A favourable examination of his genitals together with a testimony to the effect that his wife was no longer a virgin would have been sufficient to clinch the dispute in his favour. However, over-estimating the extent and limitations of his virility, De Langey offered himself up publicly to a trial by congress. It proved to be a fatal challenge.

The great day arrived. The test was to take place at the house of a certain Turpin, a steam-bath proprietor of the Faubourg Saint-Antoine. Nothing was left to chance: fifteen experts waited in attendance – five physicians, five surgeons and five matrons. Lawyers and members of the family already occupied the field, while outside a festive crowd besieged the house. The authorities responsible for public order had to be called upon to clear an entry for the protagonists.

Preceding the Marquis, who liked to stage his entrances, the Marquise arrived first, perfectly calm despite the boos of the crowd. Her husband followed shortly after: 'Langey was pro-claiming victory,' recalled an excited Tallemant, 'you would have thought he was already *in*.' Moreover, De Langey had worked out in advance each stage of the ritual, down to the tiniest details. Thus he insisted that his wife be given a hot bath, to counteract the effects of any astringents which she might have taken, and that her hair was to be left untied, to prevent her from concealing talismans which would interfere with or bewitch his performance. He would not even allow her hair to be 'coiffed with a cornet that two wives of her grandfather's kinsmen had brought with them; another cornet, belonging to the bath owner's wife, had to be used instead.' Finally the couple withdrew to bed, at which point De Langey cried out: 'Bring me two fresh eggs, that I may get her a son at the first shot' – a somewhat rash piece of optimism, considering that the trial was to last four hours:

During which time he had not the smallest stirrings where they were needed, though he did sweat plentifully such as to change his shirt twice, the drugs he had taken having inflamed him so. Next in a rage he set to praying.

'You are not here for that,' said she, and she upbraided him for the hardness with which he had always treated her, he who knew full well that he was not in any way able to perform those dues which he ought unto a wife.

In its account of this critical moment of the trial, the *Journal du Palais* portrayed the Marquise in a rather different light. Resigning herself by a pious act of self-abnegation,

> she did uncover for a time the veil of her modesty: hard necessity gave her strength: the hope of a victory though sorrowful drove her on, and while her enemy languished bereft of all vigour, she did console herself with the innocence and justness of the cause that, despite her better nature, had drawn her into so bitter an ordeal.

Whatever the actual mental state of the protagonists, the assembled company was by this time beginning to be restless:

> There was present, appointed as a matter of course, an old woman of eighty years, Madame Peze, who did get up to a hundred extravagances, from time to time going near to apprize herself of Langey's condition, and upon coming back to report to the experts: 'Tis a great pity, for he does engender naught.' At the last, his time having expired, Langey was fetched out of bed: 'I am ruined,' he cried on rising. His kinsfolk dared not to raise their eyes, and most of them did go away.

De Langey subsequently lodged a protest, demanding a second trial on the grounds that his wife had contaminated his bath with spells. His pleas fell upon deaf ears. On 8 February 1659, the High Court of Paris recorded a verdict of failure, declared the marriage null and void, ordered the Marquis to return his wife's dowry, and forbade him to remarry in the future.

The following winter there did occur at Rheims a similar case, in which the wife accorded her husband the favour of a whole night in which to prove himself. The experts waited around the fire. Many a time did he call out: 'Come! Come now!' But always it was a false alarm. The wife laughed and told them: 'Do not hurry so, for I know him well.' The experts said after that never had they laughed as much nor slept as little as on that night.

It is hardly surprising that such practices aroused the indignation of certain High Court magistrates. But the astonishing repercussions of the De Langey affair were to be the last straw.

His pride still wounded, De Langey was not a man to admit defeat. Twenty-four hours after the proclamation of the verdict confirming his impotence, he was already making a solemn declaration in the presence of two notaries to the effect that he did not consider himself impotent and reserved his right to remarry.

Having retired to her estates in Normandy, his wife – now Mademoiselle de Saint-Simon – soon found consolation in the arms of Pierre de Caumont, the Marquis de Boesse, a gentleman without fortune but of good stock, and their marriage was rapidly followed by the birth of three daughters. Meanwhile, smashing through the obstacles in his path, De Langey hastened to do the same with a certain Diane de Montault de Navailles. In actual fact the legal impediment against him was only a formality, and remarriages by men declared impotent were quite common. It would have been excusable at the time to imagine De Langey now hitched up with a thirty-year-old woman who was probably resigned to his frigidity. But the Marquis proceeded to revenge himself sevenfold upon the world, by giving his second wife seven children. 'I saw Langey at Charenton baptise his second child the other day,' noted Tallemant, 'and now that he has both son and daughter never was man so satisfied, he looked triumphant.'

With the premature death of the first Marquise de Langey in 1670, events took another dramatic turn: one of the clauses in her will contained the following explosive stipulation:

It is the wish of the testator that the unsettled lawsuit which did take place in the third chamber of appeal, between herself and M. René de Cordouan, be terminated by arrangement.

Some observers saw in this a thinly disguised acknowledgement of the 'suspicions which she had aroused in the legal profession when she did succeed in having her marriage annulled in 1659.' On 3 August 1675, in accordance with the findings of the public prosecutor, Lamoignon, the Marquis de Langey and Diane de Montault were granted their request to celebrate their marriage legally. One month later, De Langey stepped into the breach again with a civil appeal requesting the court to revoke its 1659 decision concerning his impotence.

By now it was clear that the 'reopening' of the case could be postponed no longer, however extreme the reluctance of the magistrates to put in question a previous verdict. The case was brought before the Great Chamber, to the hearings of the Thursday cause-list. But the minor nature of the appeal lodged by De Langey left it in no doubt that his real intention was to put on trial the institution of congress itself.

This was by no means the first time that the institution had been arraigned, even on the floor of a court. As early as 1640, at the time of the Costé affair, the assistant public prosecutor Jérôme Bignon had declared: 'It is necessary that we abolish these suits concerning both impotency and congress, for they are so brutish and dishonourable, that public modesty blushes nor can it endure them.' Again, in 1674, the public prosecutor Lamoignon had spoken out against the Rémy de Saint-Jallot case, in which an old man was forced into trial by congress at the injunction of the ecclesiastical judge of Coutances: 'We would hope that it were possible to abolish entirely these tests of impotency by means of congress, the which are abused so often by the Officialities.'

At about the same date, Boileau raised some laughter with a

biting satire on this theme, composed perhaps at the request of Lamoignon:

> *Never for his Impotency did a hind on heat*
> *Haul her stag from his woody retreat*
> *To appear in a court; nor ever did the judge*
> *Sully his report – when ordering conjugal zest –*
> *By recourse to a word as absurd as CONGRESS.*

Champions of congress dismissed this as mere poetic license, for never has a stag in rut promised in all solemnity to be faithful to his hind.

During the course of the eleven hearings devoted to the second De Langey case, legal quibbles flew back and forth concerning the unavoidable dilemma posed by the 1659 verdict. The dilemma which was paralysing the course of justice was perfectly genuine: were the judges to revoke the earlier decision or to let it stand, they would in either case be acting in breach of the law. For if De Langey was in fact impotent, what was to be done about the decision which had just legalised his second marriage? What of his children? On the other hand, if he was not impotent, then his first marriage was legitimate, in which case not only was he now guilty of bigamy, but in perpetrating this crime he had enjoyed the complicity of the authorities.

Contrary to expectations, the case started off badly for De Langey. His lawyer, Pageau, tried to remind the court that the physical attributes or natural state of an individual were subject to the law of estoppel. Verdicts were only binding for contracts based on a conscious act of will, and which could therefore lend themselves to the interpretation of the judges. But were these same judges entitled to apply the law to human nature itself, their knowledge of which was surely so inadequate? Pageau argued in vain, for this philosophy was difficult to reconcile with the spirit of seventeenth-century jurisprudence. In matters of impotence, it did not triumph completely until the nineteenth century.

Thus the De Langey case ended in a patched-up compromise. The court confirmed the 1659 decision and deemed as unacceptable the appeal lodged by De Langey. At the same time, stirred by the impassioned speech of the public prosecutor Lamoignon, the court surrendered completely under the weight of irreconcilable legal paradox, and abolished at a stroke the whole institution of trial by congress. By a capital decree of 18 February 1677, 'the court, acceding to the conclusions of the public prosecutor to the King, henceforth forbids all judges, including those of the Officialities, to order trial by congress in marital disputes.'

A universal chorus of praise now rose up around Chrétien François de Lamoignon, the champion of modesty. Three years later, Lamoignon confirmed his vocation by publishing a *Plea concerning congress*, a brilliant synthesis of the main arguments against this practice. However, although banished from the courts, trial by congress proved more difficult to eliminate from public memory. During the next century and a half, there was hardly a writer who did not dwell with morbid complacency upon the misfortunes of the Marquis de Langey. The pretexts for this were always the purest: prior to 1789 it was a question of extolling the virtues of Lamoignon and the High Court of Paris; thereafter it was the need to denounce the obscenities of the *Ancien Régime*.

In 1734, the magistrate Bouhier even reopened the controversy by attempting to rehabilitate trial by congress, in his audacious *Treatise on the Measures in Force in France for determining Impotency in Men*. Sailing against the current of the time, he tried to argue that congress furnished the ultimate proof, provided it could be stripped of the abuses which had thrown it into disrepute in the past. According to Bouhier, the trial had all too often been unjustly imposed or conducted in a

deplorable fashion: no effort was made to carry out the
mandatory preliminary visit to the wife; the husband was often
refused exemption from the trial although his wife was known
or discovered to be a virgin; congress had usurped the mandatory three-year cohabitation period; trials were conducted
hastily in a matter of hours, and so on. Trial by congress would
from now on be considered as a lifeline held out to a drowning
man, not as a noose held around his neck. Bouhier's work
inspired the jurist Fromageot to an indignant if thoroughly dull
reply, and a similar flatness characterised the chaste counter-
attack in Gayot de Pitival's *Famous Cases*.

It would nevertheless be a mistake to consider the abolition
of congress and this subsequent rearguard action as indicating
a radical departure from the hotch-potch of obscene practices
which were so characteristic of the period as a whole. On the
contrary, these new elements were grafted onto an underlying
controversy, partly philosophical and partly juridical, which
was as old as the institution of congress itself.

It is hardly surprising that so extraordinary an institution
should have provoked furious controversy. As early as 1577,
the arguments were sparked off by the case of De Bray, who
was seen to botch trial by congress three times in succession
before declining the offer of a fourth attempt. In 1580 Antoine
Hotman, the counsel for the defence of this eminent person-
age, drafted a factum of the case which was loaded with
scathing references to inconsistencies in the system. A year later
he published an anonymous treatise *Of the Dissolution of
Marriages by the Impotency and Frigidity of the Husband or
Wife*, in which trial by congress was closely scrutinised but in a
more general context, since Hotman made no allusion to his
unfortunate client. The success of this dogmatic survey – it in
fact ran to a second edition – provoked an immediate reaction
from none other than the lawyer, Etienne Pasquier, who had

conducted the case for the defence of Marie de Corbie against De Bray. Moreover, in his factum he unreservedly declared himself a fervent apologist of trial by congress, and stated without any scruples that 'there is modesty in such an act', and that it was 'the clearest means of proof that exists or that could exist.'

The same beliefs fired the lawyer Sébastien Roulliard when he loudly proclaimed the infallibility and solemnity of trial by congress, in a curious capitulary published at the very beginning of the seventeenth century. It is true that this jurist was writing at the behest of D'Argenton, to whom the judges of the time had not even granted the 'favour' of a trial by congress to refute the accusations of impotence levelled at him.

In 1610, the controversy was given a new impetus by the case of an unlucky husband, whose misadventures inspired Tagereau to compose an erudite *Discourse on the Impotence of Men and Women*. Here, the forensic procedures, the appraisals by experts and the trial itself are depicted as an obnoxious conspiracy dreamed up for the sole purpose of ruining men.

Apart from this handful of specialist works on the subject, an endless stream of criticism appeared from all quarters. Physicians and surgeons (Paré, Guillemeau, Venette), jurists (Anne Robert, the public prosecutors Bignon and Lamoignon), theologians (Fevret, Sainte-Beuve) and men of letters (Boileau) all united with one voice to condemn trial by congress. A confused babel of arguments and suggestions kept alive a controversy which turned upon two basic themes: modesty and inefficiency.

All these writings primarily and universally condemned the cynical premeditation and execution of the act of love 'in cold blood' before witnesses:

What is more obscene than this congress which gives permission to witness private parts mingle with private parts, and flesh dissolve into flesh? What is more filthy and unseemly than to couple in front of all and sundry?

It is a law that does offend modesty; it is too harsh and injurious to the husband, whereby he has to make visible to others those parts that Nature has hid with such care.

But if congress be shameful for the man, it is far more so for the woman, since with infamy and unseemliness she must make a show of herself, and reveal her shame, exposing herself to a filthy and immodest nudity, yielding herself to the hands and eyes of another all that Nature has taken care to conceal from others.

History was seen as profusely illustrated with edifying examples:

The woman that is made public, by stripping herself of all shame in such an act, thereafter does closet and hide herself. Before, when there were neither houses nor buildings, people still sought out caves and dark places to perform such acts.

[Out of modesty] Lycurgus had ordained that the newly-wed man should not visit his wife but at night, and then surreptitiously, and in fear and shame that he be noticed by any member of his household. [This is, of course, a false interpretation; the Spartan legislator was attempting by this law to establish the preponderance of homosexual over heterosexual relations – the latter were tolerated only in the interests of a rising birth rate.]

In Ancient Rome, the husband lay not at all with his wife during the day, but only at night, and then without lights.

And it was salutary to ponder the lessons of nature:

The pleasures of the bed are brutish, and transient, and after practising them we do set to repenting of them. Let us not then imitate those lascivious beasts and throw ourselves with vacated bodies and sightless eyes upon the promiscuous venery of the flesh.

Again, all animals have not the 'shamelessness of dogs . . .'

Even frogs, that are vile and base creatures, do hold it in horror to embrace during the day, and await the fall of night before coupling.

It is a certain fact that between elephants there was never and is never committed adultery, and that they do never mate except in a privy retired place, all removed from the main tracks and from other company; not do they return to the troop after mating, unless they have first washed and as if purified themselves in brisk and running water. How then do men not blush? With what complacency then, and with what eye, can physicians, surgeons and others so named, watch so infamous and loathsome a spectacle?

For Tagereau, the elephants' admirable modesty was equalled only by that of camels.

The partisans of trial by congress were not even allowed to console themselves with its efficiency; for love is capricious, independent, and the enemy of daylight. It does not stand to attention at the order of a judge. Our hands, feet, eyes and tongues all obey our wishes, but the sexual organs follow only those impulses generated by the complicity of two minds. Moreover, congress was regarded as resting upon an untenable proposition: 'How can you expect,' exclaimed Tagereau, 'that a man relentlessly hounded [into trial by congress] by his wife can possibly be able to join himself to her in the act of love?'

Advocates of congress focused their arguments around an elementary but solid principle: because of its perhaps somewhat brutal realism, the trial was the only efficient means of detecting and making harmless the impotent man who profanes the sacrament of marriage by violating it with impunity, concealed as he is behind the veil of its sacred mystery. Congress was perhaps evil, but it is the lesser evil.

Violating all the taboos, the lawyer Bernard even went so far as to praise a certain beauty which, according to him, surrounded the ceremony of congress. Unique of its kind, this audacious declaration of principle seemed inspired by a sort of lyricism. Lost in the higher spheres of contemplation, Bernard addressed himself to Guillaume Desmaret, who had just been condemned to trial by congress by a verdict of 20 January 1587:

The judge invites you to congress, to make essay of a brave and lusty love in the soft bed that is raised with fine ticking filled out with feathers; wherein you will find lying a young girl of beauteous excellence, in the first flower of her youth, that awaits only the embraces of her dear spouse; you will see her eyes shining with a tremulous gleam, you will see youth lambent with desire, you will be aroused to love's battle by an infinity of kissing and colling, you will be given free rein to bite her crimson lips and leave love's bites upon them, and to kiss her marble throat, and with an impatient hand to kindle those fires of love that late had died down all languishing. There Venus has her seat, and all the gentle cupids, and there reclines voluptuous delight incarnate. But if the pleasant kisses and the lascivious blandishments naught avail in firing Titius, if those parts of the body that ought to sustain all the vigour of love are then still cold, without sensation, spiritless, languishing, cooler than ice, and if they do not show forth themselves and stand erect, if they do not water the garden of Venus and warm it with a rosy balm, but recede into the body in shame, and if the arms that are entwined each in each do not tighten in the strenuous lists of pleasure, if the body be all slack, and the breasts that demand to be clasped each to each in the bonds of love do disappoint all good intentions, then there is surely no hope that Titius may prove himself a man, and no assurance of there being issue by such a marriage. In vain will Titius then demand reprieves, in vain will he long to find out some hiding place and seek the obscurity of night.

In addition to this erotic vein in the writings of the time, there was another kind of pornography which, despite appearances, led to the very roots of the institution itself. The flamboyant eroticism which emerged in the sermons of a whole tribe of misogynous preachers has obvious affinities with the spirit of congress itself. By mounting the pulpit to fulminate against everything that did not give off an odour of perfect purity and godliness, these bigoted orators were part of a tradition which had given birth to the institution of congress. In other words, the sermon was to the preacher precisely what congress had been to the authorities. Both constituted privileged areas, in which an obsession with sexuality was apparent. The subject of female nudity was one of the great ecclesiastical specialities of the seventeenth century. It appears and reappears indefatigably in the writings of Polman, Boileau, Juvernay, Bouvignes, and others. On the surface it took the form of repellent reactionary tendencies, but behind the façade of blundering, puritanical misogyny there lurked a confused libido, a mixture of excitement and despair:

God contemns nudity in women because he is Cleanness incarnate, the Demon worships it because he is polluted; God contemns nudity because it is the symbol of our Fall; the Fiend loves it because it is the mark of his triumph; God contemns nudity because it is the cause and the consequence of Sin, the Demon loves it because it is the visible proof of our misery and because it uncovers at once our destitution and our crime . . .

But the attention of preachers was to crystallise far more precisely around the subject of the female breast, which seventeenth-century fashion brought into favour and exhibited boldly. At the beginning of the century, a war was declared against 'the uncovering of breasts and teats'. As early as 1617, an anonymous pamphlet entitled *The Courtesan Revealed* denounced the 'lascivious' woman who, 'like to those hags [witches], uncovers her bosom and her nipples to lure to her whomsoever she pleases, and having thus cast a spell with her beauty does make them loathsome and infamous.'

This was a theme upon which the canon Jean Polman was to play magnificent variations, in a collection of sermons entitled *The Canker: On the Covering of Female Breasts*:

The Fashionables, those carnal progeny of Babylon, do throw lascivious looks upon the whiteness of a revealed bosom; they do aim unclean thoughts at the cleavage between those two mounds of flesh; they house villainous desires in the hollow of that naked breast; they do fasten their lusts upon those swelling mounds; they find a resting place for their concupiscence in this bed and lair of dugs, where they can commit bawdiness in their minds.

Father Louis de Bouvignes proved to be equally concerned for the salvation of the poor wretches who let themselves be seduced by the charms of a pair of breasts:

'I am confused,' he confides to an imaginary courtesan, 'when I watch you uncover thus your arms, and show your throat, and prostitute your breast which is unceasingly lashed by the lascivious looks of men.'

And Father de Barry compared this 'vanity of the breast' to a 'plague-bearer and a venom which does empoison from afar when one casts one's eyes upon it, or when one touches it.' He imagined that breasts emanated an incurable evil.

In the case of Pierre Juvernay and Jacques Boileau, this plague begins to take on dramatic proportions. These two ecclesiastics saw breasts everywhere: at the 'holie communion', where priests revealed themselves to be for the most part 'simpletons, sharpers [hypocrites], flatterers' and accomplices in immodesty, at processions, and even during church collections, where 'one does see female collectors so slovenly that you would take them to be actresses, farcers and masqueraders.' And the height of indecency, for Juvernay, was the sight of society women who had taken to wearing 'a cross or image of the Holy Spirit hung at their breasts . . . they would do better to wear in that place the image of a toad or a crow, since these animals too take their pleasures among the ordures.'

Jacques Boileau, who devoted an entire pamphlet to *The Abuse of the Nakedness of Breasts* (1675), was prey to a similar phobia: 'It is not solely in private houses, at balls, in the public walks, in the Ladies' Ruelles [salons], that women do parade their naked breasts: there are those who, with a most astounding boldness, come to insult Jesus Christ at the very feet of the altar.' It was in this way that they were considered most dangerous to the souls of men who, according to Boileau, are 'innocent and righteous' but also 'faltering in virtue'. Some moralists took delight in pointing out the disappointments which befell slovenly coquettes: 'Look at this common stale [prostitute],' exclaimed Monsieur de la Serre [a lay convert to the ranks of the most bigoted preachers], 'she has no beauty beyond that of her breasts, the which she brazenly parades as if the rest of her body were for hire or to sell. Oh! how ashamed must she feel at the end of the day, when she sees herself forced to close up her shop without having found a single admirer for her merchandise.'

The tragic consequences of the 'uncovering of breasts and teats' even sent a shiver of sadism through the good Father de Barry:

> Breasts are not after all two small muck-hills covered in snow, but two pounds of flesh which do cost a great deal to the foolish women who bare them and believe themselves thereby to be the more beautiful and the more pleasing ... For their bosoms become cold from prolonged nudity, their swellings shrink down and do sometimes remain thus, when lo and behold death carries them off.

> A young lady of three-and-twenty years did die of a sudden: the doctors had her opened up and could find no cause for death other than a cold bosom. I have seen another die who was but seven or eight years old, but who had already been accustomed to having an uncovered breast; my belief was that the cold had seized this little uncovered chest and that God, in his bounty, had taken her early from this world, to relieve her of the temptation and opportunity to continue in earthly vanities.

Such preoccupations were an aspect of the psychological context within which the trials for impotence evolved. This sanctified pornography, the need to define women in a debilitating and marginal role, the trial by congress itself and the institution of the medical visit all merged and reinforced each other. The ecclesiastical judge who prescribed trial by congress and the orator who condemned the breast were united in a practice whose purpose was to maintain them in intellectual contact with the flesh.

This is the fundamental meaning behind the trial of the sexually impotent. The institution only survived through three centuries thanks to the ambiguous indulgence of the Church, and its abuse of its privilege in the ossified society of the *Ancien Régime*. Thus it is not surprising that the French Revolution, by making civil law triumph over canon law in matrimonial affairs, should have brought about a temporary decline in marital lawsuits.

Conclusion
The myth of virility

There is no sense in which the impotence trials of the *Ancien Régime* can strictly be compared with modern lawsuits for impotence. The Revolution in 1789, or to be more precise the legislation of 1792, initiated a complete change of style. Marriage became a civil contract and the divorce laws were instituted. The temporary abolition of divorce in France, from 1824 to 1884, did not fundamentally affect this transformation. In the majority of cases, separations on the grounds of impotence were conducted outside ecclesiastical jurisdiction, and were therefore spared the obscene and impassioned procedures which in the past had aroused the unhealthy imagination of magistrates and provoked the ridicule of the public. From now on, the institution of divorce by mutual consent or on the grounds of incompatibility constituted a powerful safety valve, added to which the temporary return to a policy of indissolubility, even for cases of impotence, served to contain the problem – if in a rather radical fashion. From this point of view the nineteenth century was the age of sagacity and sobriety, especially given the fact that the *code civil* took no account of impotence, concerning which all judges were unanimous: it was not in itself a reason for divorce.

However, this rational attitude was superficial, and beneath it there existed the elements of a reaction which was to increase in strength towards the end of the century and blossom in the twentieth century.

On 20 September 1792, the legislative Assembly, deeming that the existence of any indissoluble contract was in flagrant contradiction to the free exercise of individual liberty, legalised divorce. This measure, which had been demanded for a long time by numerous jurists and *philosophes*, was all the more revolutionary and anti-clerical in that those articles concerning divorce by mutual consent and on the grounds of incompatibility made the law astonishingly liberal.

But these modern, if not avant-garde, provisions often concealed the most reactionary mentality when it came to putting theory into practice. The lawyer Garnier was in this respect one of the spirits of the age, and his *Code du Divorce*, published shortly after the law of September 1792, is a concrete embodiment of that spirit.

The exegetics to which Garnier was inspired by the notion of incompatibility of temperament had strong elements of fanaticism and intolerance inherited from the *Ancien Régime*. For among the causes of divorce on the grounds of incompatibility, hatred of the Revolution occupied a prominent place. From the ecclesiastic heaping anathema upon the unbeliever to the revolutionary denouncing the enemies of the Revolution, the gulf was not so very wide. It was a relatively simple matter to substitute one religion for another.

Garnier's intolerance was as strong when it came to resolving a certain number of problems relating to 'dissoluteness of morals', and in his account of sodomy he joins the great tradition of classical preachers.

Moreover, by heaping anathema upon the victims of venereal diseases, Garnier showed himself to be far more intolerant than his predecessors during the *Ancien Régime*. Similarly, he argued that sterility was an irrefutable reason for divorce. Though now there was certainly no longer any question of breeding in the spirit of the Book of Genesis, the nation did have to be repopulated. It is hardly surprising, in these circumstances, that Garnier should have included impotence among the grounds for divorce, and it is striking the extent to which his arguments here rely upon a simple restatement of the classical themes, adapted to the ideological shift produced by the Revolution.

In fact the divorce laws of 1792 passed over in silence the question of impotence. The problem had stained the reputation of courts during the *Ancien Régime*, and the revolutionary assemblies were reluctant to inherit the burden. A few years later, the modest silences and innuendoes of the *code civil* were also to become a breeding ground for misunderstandings and controversy throughout the nineteenth century.

The embarrassed silence of the *code civil* on the question of impotence unfortunately left the door wide open to all kinds of interpretations and exegetics. Originally, the committee responsible for drawing up the *code* had anticipated a bill rejecting 'the allegation of natural or accidental impotence in a husband'. In the words of the court reporter, it was 'difficult and scandalous to prove'. But this bill was itself rejected by the Council of State, the mere allusion to impotence being found to be inopportune and scabrous. Thus bourgeois puritanism, a determining feature of the society produced by the Revolution, pursued a policy of moral austerity to the point of obliterating the problem.

But this choice placed the legislators in a self-contradictory position. For the *code* recognised elsewhere the repudiation of paternity in cases of accidental impotence. It was strange, to say the least, that the law should on the one hand take no account of allegations of impotence, while on the other making an exception for the rule of *pater est quem*. It was owing to this central ambiguity that the problem of impotence was soon to resurface.

The reasons for the legal differentiation between natural impotence and accidental impotence were simple. The First Consul explained them at length during a debate of the Council of State:

Provision in law must be limited to cases of accidental impotence. It is not possible to recognise natural impotence; in the first place, the legislator should not attempt to penetrate the secrets which nature has concealed; in the second place, his silence on the matter is in the interest of the children. Accidental impotence, on the other hand, is a physical fact concerning which there can be no mistake, hence the legislator may not ignore it.

It is worth adding that the jurists were receptive to the far more generous diagnostic of accidental impotence. But underlying everything, two fundamental social principles of the new bourgeois order were confronting each other. On one hand, it was important to protect at all costs the sacrosanct rights of property, by preventing inheritances from falling into the wrong hands. A repudiation of paternity supported by an admission of natural impotence would be meaningless by reason of its purely subjective character, but the same repudiation would be validated by an avowal of accidental impotence, which has an objective reality. On the other hand, it was important to reduce to a minimum the number of socially disruptive illegitimate offspring.

In fact, in the absence of specific articles and texts on the subject of impotence, nineteenth-century jurists elaborated, with a great show of exegetical paraphernalia, doctrinal systems to which some of them even attempted to lend the authority of the law. The urge to integrate sexual incapacity within a juridical framework was undoubtedly very strong. By invoking the question of an error in the choice of partner, the scope of accidental impotence was increased and given a far more solid foundation. Article 146 of the *code civil* already specified that there could be no marriage without consent. Expanding this clause, article 180 added that, where there was error in the choice of partner, the marriage could be contested by the partner who had been misled. The majority of jurists proclaimed their attachment to this doctrine. It wasa a partial solution, but a solution nonetheless.

The attitude of forensic doctors was even more recalcitrant, in some cases to the point of ferocity. At the beginning of the nineteenth century, Dr Fodéré, an expert on the subject, declared that the essential conditions for a marriage to be valid were consent and the capacity to fulfil the conjugal duty. According to him, an error in the choice of partner – and consequent invalidation of the union – occurred when there was a mistake as to sex, impotence or 'onset of some hideous disease'. But to put on the same level 'error as to sex' and impotence was in itself an improper bias. Moreover, Fodéré did not even attempt to establish a realistic distinction between accidental and natural impotence. As for the allusion to 'hideous disease', it is hardly reassuring to find jumbled together in this category the 'various stages of imbecility', Saint Vitus's dance, somnambulism, haemoptysis, bronchial and cardiac asthma and aneurism.

Such intransigence far surpassed the severity of the earlier legislation. The religious impediments decreed by canon law were merely replaced by utilitarian interdictions better suited to the spirit of the time. All the above ailments are hereditary, and Fodéré claimed 'to know of no other means of ridding Europe of them than by preventing these kinds of people from marrying.' Today we have a clearer idea as to the logical outcome of a racial ideology founded upon such criteria of selection. Fodéré's preventative argument could fool nobody, and his nostalgic invocation of Sparta is all that was needed to reveal the true nature of his argument: 'In this city, a happily combined stock of people seemed to add a new infusion of strength and majesty to human nature; nothing was so beautiful, and nothing so pure, as the blood of the Spartans.' The exaltation of virility through a condemnation and exclusion of the impotent individual combined with a paean of praise to blood, in an apparently coherent argument, contains a confession which merits some thought.

Half a century later, the manual of forensic medicine by Briand and Chaude, although far more lenient about the state of health required of marriage partners, is no less intransigent in its position on impotence. From the outset, error in the choice of partner, which was originally meant to cover mistaken sexuality, is extended to include not only 'accidental, manifest and pre-marital' impotence, but also 'natural impotence, and those cases where it is so manifest that it cannot be held in doubt.'

But these isolated attitudes, the heritage of a recent but buried past, could not challenge the new legal spirit. In reality, male frigidity, that invisible form of impotence which for centuries had confused jurists, physicians and theologians, was finally banished from the courts, and impotence trials became extremely rare during the nineteenth century.

However, this attitude was not in any way inspired by an elevated conception of marriage. It derived rather from the bourgeois puritanism which triumphed during this period and which sacrificed the interests of the individual to the imperatives of public morality: 'If private interests must suffer,' noted a decree of 10 March 1858, 'it is justifiable to impose such a sacrifice in the broader interests of public order and morals.'

Scruples of this kind did not unduly trouble the ecclesiastical courts during the nineteenth century, which, mindful of their evangelical purpose, perpetuated the traditions of preceding centuries. In fact, the attempts of civil courts to be discreet in matters of impotence had no effect upon the obtrusive procedures still in force in the ecclesiastical courts. Although the latter only dealt with a limited number of cases after civil legislation rejected impotence as a reason for annulment, the basic principles of canon law persisted in their traditional form, and the few impotence trials which were referred to the

Church courts still followed a procedure which had hardly changed since the eighteenth century. The only change in the procedural system was its increased centralisation: all trials were now submitted to Rome for approval. This shift towards the summit of power was made possible only by the appreciable decline in the number of trials.

There exists a very thorough documentation on those nineteenth-century impotence trials held in Church courts, thanks to a directive issued by Pius IX in 1858. This document is in effect an exhaustive inventory of eighteenth-century texts and practices. It shows that cross-examinations of the partners were still ordered with a view to extracting the fullest possible confession. The Pope laid down the main guidelines for these interrogations in a non-restrictive manner, and to judge by the suggested pattern of questions, the test continued to be a thinly disguised and indecent inquisition into the private lives of the faithful:

During the night of the nuptial celebrations, did the couple lie in the same house and in the same bed? Did they attend to their conjugal duties spontaneously and willingly? Did they consummate the marriage?

Did [non-consummation] occur as a result of the excessive narrowness of the wife's vulva, or was it caused by the excessive size of the husband's member, or by his feebleness, such that there was not the least erection, even of a momentary nature?

To which relatives, friends or neighbours did the spouse in question confide that the marriage had not been consummated? He or she is to name them individually. [Here the *septima manus* has been revived.]

Next followed the examination of the witnesses: first the parents or relatives, followed by the servants, the neighbours, and so on. The outlines of the inquisition would now become increasingly clear: 'Does the witness know the couple? does he know whether they have lain together? whether they have consummated their marriage? . . .'

When it came to the medical examination of the genitals,

there were no scruples over subtle distinctions between natural and accidental impotence. The example of civil legislation in such matters had done nothing to shake the conviction of Church courts that non-consummation remained the sole criterion, whatever the causes of the impotence from which it proceeded. It is worth noting in this connection that the proof of erection was never officially repudiated, and one ambiguous phrase in the pontifical directive of 1858 seems even to have implicitly authorised it. 'It is necessary,' advised the Holy Father, 'to verify whether the penis is capable of a prompt erection which can last the time necessary for the achievement of coitus.'

As for the medical examination of the woman, its procedures were systematised and no longer subject to any restriction or moral scruple. Two midwives were to observe and palpate the woman and then draw up a report of their findings. Two doctors were to read the document and interpret it. Thus, those who had seen the woman in question said nothing, and those who had not seen her gave an opinion. But it was believed that this system preserved dignity and spared modesty.

The directive of 1858 underlines once more the inquisitorial nature of trials in the Church courts. And yet, for the whole of the nineteenth century the ecclesiastical courts, in France at least, were plunged into a kind of torpor as a result of the intransigence of the civil courts. This torpor would seem to have ended with the reinstatement of divorce in 1884 and the covert rehabilitation of impotence as a reason for separation. It was about this date that the canonical reaction that has continued into the twentieth century was born.

From the end of the nineteenth century there was a change of direction, and impotence gradually re-emerged from its obscurity. Officially, this reversal did not involve any rehabilitation of the practices and preconceptions of former times.

Indeed, until very recently impotence was banished from the
courts, which were endlessly reminded in 'preambles' that 'it
does not constitute grounds for the annulment of a marriage.'

However, behind this puritanical façade inherited from the
nineteenth century a doctrine was slowly evolving which
served to reinstate the basic principles of the older law. Admittedly, considerable care was taken to avoid any overt accusations of impotence. It was preferable to use the term
'non-consummation', which did not imply *a priori* any sexual
incapacity, but which had the added advantage of implicating
the accused more easily, because it presupposed a deliberate act
of will. Within such a perspective divorce merely replaced
annulment, and non-consummation became grounds for
separation by placing the fault on the side of the partner who
chose not to consummate the marriage.

As for the old hobby-horse of nineteenth-century jurists,
error in the choice of partner, this was hardly ever invoked. It
was not until the ruling of 20 November 1958 that, thanks to
an error of this kind, annulment once again came to prevail
over divorce in matters of impotence.

At the beginning of the century, however, only 'identity of
sex' categorically resulted in annulment. But the three main
incriminatory pretexts of the modern period – 'identity of sex',
'error' and 'maltreatment' – all serve the same purpose: to
disgrace the impotent husband or wife.

'Illicit sexual practices' inspired a good deal of curiosity and
oratorical excesses. In 1894, the court of appeal of Nîmes
turned its attention to the case of a husband who, 'instead of
fulfilling his conjugal duties', was guilty 'of having substituted
illicit, shameful and unnatural practices, libidinous caresses
and fondlings which no honest woman could support.' No
doubt the judges refrained from prying directly into 'those
secrets of the marriage bed, upon which it would be immodest,
let alone impossible, to bring to bear the investigations of a

court enquiry.' But for all that the couple, during the hearings of the counsel chamber, had cast 'a sufficient light upon the lamentable struggles in which they were locked', and the judges did not seem reluctant to dwell upon subjects they were forbidden to take any notice of. Thus we learn soon after that 'the lady D. is clearly still a virgin', that 'her husband has made every effort to rid her of this state', that 'the scratch-marks left by nails' which the surgeons found 'are the fruit of fondlings and caresses in which the husband indulged and which his wife endured, even if she did not actively provoke them.'

In some cases the refinements of scabrous detail are quite astonishing. One of the reasons adduced by the Lyons Court of Appeal for its ruling of 28 May 1956 was that 'the marriage of X and Y was only consummated seven months after its celebration, on the bold initiative of the wife, and in the course of which she acted courageously and generously; this was the last of their sexual relations in the complete sense of the term, the others being unsuccessful and satisfactory only to the husband.'

Scandalous fabrications of this kind could take on tragic dimensions, as in one very recent ruling of the Departmental Court of Dieppe. Here the fabrication was all the more cruel in that it concerned the 'crime' of a seventy-year-old man who in all probability wanted merely to think of himself as still in his twenties. After six months of marriage, Mme N. claimed 'that her husband demonstrated a voracious sexual appetite, treating his wife as an object of his free, total and absolute disposal.' The husband's testimony is rather touching: 'I enjoyed myself whenever I had the urge to enjoy myself, and I did what it is only normal to do when one is married.' Unmoved, however, the judges publicly criticised these final convulsions of a fading sexuality, and in terms bordering on the sadistic they denounced this husband whose behaviour has degenerated from tenderness to indecency and the most extreme bestiality, who cannot go near his wife without trying to caress and embrace her or lift up her skirt to fondle her, and who pesters her repeatedly each day with his attentions, covering her body with kisses . . .

This new propensity for salacious detail was only one aspect of a general return to the style and spirit of the *Ancien Régime*.

Another aspect of this regression was confession extorted by means of formal enquiries, and often in an improper manner. In the ruling of the Departmental Court of Grenoble in 1958, it was in defiance of medical ethics that a doctor's certificate was added to the file of the case, in which 'Dr R. attested that since 1952 he had been treating X for sexual impotence, and declared that the condition of the latter was stationary.' A verdict of the Departmental Court of the Seine in 1961 even noted that

if the proof of a deliberate refusal to consummate a marriage is difficult to establish by means of an enquiry, it is not beyond the bounds of possibility to discover in the testimony of the witnesses certain facts from which the behaviour of the partners in respect of consummation may be deduced.

This was no less than a lay form of the *septima manus*.

From 1880 onwards, however, the harsh ethos of law manuals and the imperatives of forensic medicine had come to the fore, and killed off all remaining scruples. It is true that medical examinations were not compulsory, but the refusal to submit to an examination 'could be taken into account and, to a certain extent, used to corroborate other evidence contributed to the case.' By 1924, there no longer existed even the illusion of a free choice in the matter of medical examinations. One husband, widowed at the birth of his seventh child, was subsequently taken to court in 1924 by his second wife on a charge of impotence. The civil court of Pont-l'Evêque confined itself to noting 'the existence of certain difficulties in the conjugal relations' of the couple, and ordered that the husband undergo a medical examination of the genitals.

The setting-up of an apparatus for cases of 'identity of sex' was perfected at the beginning of the twentieth century, and enshrined by the court of Douai. By returning a verdict against a Mme G., which was formulated in the most offensive terms, the judges seem to have wished to revive the most severe traditions and principles of the eighteenth century: 'Whereas,' runs this verdict, 'Mme G., being possessed of neither vagina nor ovaries, although having breasts and a clitoris, is hereby deemed to be in reality not a woman but an incomplete personality, upon whom the law did never wittingly impose union with a man . . .' The judges were not content merely to give a ruling. The 'inconsistency' of the unfortunate woman was next subjected to moral considerations which were elaborated upon at her expense:

Considering that she has never had her periods, she could not be unaware of the abnormality of this fact or of its prejudicial implications from a matrimonial point of view . . . and given that she entirely disregarded her physiological state, she has at the very least committed a grave act of negligence, if not an offence whose consequences she has no right to complain at having to suffer . . .

Another pretext for incrimination, the refusal to accomplish the conjugal duty, could be treated as a serious offence and just grounds for divorcing a husband, provided that it proceeded from a deliberate act of will. Officially, impotence as such was therefore not in question, and jurisprudence provides only relatively straightforward individual cases: either of a husband who, not having received the whole amount of the dowry, touches his wife only with repugnance and declares 'that she stinks from head to toe', or of a drunkard who prefers solitary vices to conjugal pleasures.

A certain 'Mme P.G.' complained of the scornful abstention of her husband from his conjugal duties. The latter for his part immediately cited the 'fierce resistance of his wife'. However the correspondence of the couple, which left no doubt as to their mutual affection, made his allegations implausible. The husband was condemned by the court of first instance. He appealed, and attributed his sexual passivity 'to the weakness of his temperament' which made all sexual relations impossible for him. Unfortunately, medical certificates testified to his physical normality and probable virility. His sexual abstention was therefore deemed to be voluntary and insulting to his wife.

Clearly, it no longer paid to be virile. This paradox clouded the issues and undermined the basis of each trial. Henceforth neither the offence of abstention nor the misfortune of impotence retained any credibility. How could a verdict of the Court of Appeal be taken seriously, when a divorce was granted and the blame attributed exclusively to the husband, because he unfortunately 'failed to allege the existence of any physical impediment on his part which might justify his abstention'?

One major step backwards into reaction was taken with the condemnation of a potent but sterile wife in the Court of Appeal. Doubtless 'Mme. S.' had concealed from her future husband a 'physical malformation which constituted an obstacle to marriage.' But she subsequently underwent an operation which 'restored a normal physical conformation', though without any guarantee that she could have children. The appeal court of Algiers, in 1947, and the High Court of Appeal in 1951, both ruled that this operation, despite its partial success, 'was not sufficient to efface the injurious behaviour' of the woman's original act of concealment. Here, for the first time, sterility was subjected to penalties – an ominous precedent.

In its details, the schema of accusation proliferated. Illicit and contraceptive sexual practices, the premarital dissimulation of a state of impotence, the refusal to submit to a course of appropriate therapy, these were all integrated in turn within the broad spectrum of injurious behaviour and offence.

Henceforth, judges were noted for increasingly extreme verdicts. On 12 May 1958, the appeal court of Nancy even accepted confession on the part of the accused as formal proof of impotence. This amounted to an admission, two centuries after Bouhier, of the impossibility of resolving such cases other than on a basis of conjecture. By the same token it encouraged collusion between the litigants and favoured a form of disguised divorce by mutual consent, at a time when the latter was still prohibited.

The lamentable failure of the civil courts to find a juridical solution to the problem of impotence in the course of this century may account for the reaction in the sphere of canon law.

The reduction of the sexual act to the status of a pure juridical concept can be seen as the basis of the canonical reaction of the twentieth century. Probed, analysed and dissected, the sexual life of the married couple became the object of a systematic re-examination whose avowed aim was to provide the Church with a solid basis for intervention, supervision and coercion. The sexual act was fossilized within a juridical structure of constraint. The canonical terminology is astonishingly candid at this point:

> Conjugal duty: by this expression is understood the marital act as required by law of a spouse at the request of his or her partner (canon 1051, para. 1).

This means in effect that each party undertakes to render to the other, at his or her request, the *debitum conjugale*, and acquires the right to demand in turn the identical service (canon 1081, para. 1).

There exists a perfect equality of rights between husband and wife: the one or the other may take the initiative, whereupon the other is obliged to comply (canon 1111).

To this increasingly absolutist conception of the conjugal duty, there corresponded a more and more extensive definition of impotence. The pontifical ruling of 17 August 1920 submitted the validity of the sexual act to three conditions: 'A sufficient erection of the penis, its penetration into the vagina of the wife, and a veritable ejaculation of semen.' The novelty was not so much in the combination of these three traditional prerequisites as in their increasingly restrictive interpretation.

For centuries, theologians with troubled consciences had debated the crucial problem: how far should penetration proceed, and at what point does ejaculation become canonically valid?

It was only at the beginning of the twentieth century that a doctrinal position was formulated concerning this question, by Cardinal Gasparri, the intransigence of which was to cause the ruin of several husbands accused of impotence despite their having fathered a whole family of children. In a *Tractatus de matrimonio*, which has been reprinted several times since, Gasparri stated that *copula matrimonialis* was the total intromission of the penis into the vagina, the sole legitimate receptacle for semen. This doctrine rested upon an evangelical imperative: *erunt duo in carne una*. Translated into plain language, this meant that all semen scattered around the female orifice did not count as part of the carnal pact, and that any conception resulting from this accidental and canonically heterodox impregnation could in no sense validate the marriage. From this doctrine, which was enshrined by a ruling of Pius XII on 12 February 1941, came the annulment by the court of Rome of a number of fertile marriages. It was also the root of the bitter controversy which arose between Julien Demey and the *Ami du Clergé*.

Julien Demey argued that, according to the terms of canon 1013, procreation constituted the sole end of marriage. Physical satisfactions were no more than a secondary aim. Above all, he argued that it was the situation of children born from an imperfect copulation that threw a sinister light upon Gasparri's doctrine:

From this point of view, the annulment of the marriage would constitute nothing less than a crime against childhood, deliberately perpetrated by the ecclesiastical authorities. What possible respect can we expect children to retain for their parents as soon as they learn of the debate instituted on the subject of their procreation?

Even worse: 'we have seen cases which involved the summoning as witnesses of minors whose own procreation was the subject of the proceedings.'

Another aspect of the problem was how to prove that conception had occurred outside the normal pattern of consummation. This was very simple, according to the *Ami du Clerge*, for in such cases 'the hymen remains intact'. If this is so, one may well ask how – or from where – the child might be born!

The theory of imperfect coitus made nonsense of the rule of *pater est quem* which had hitherto been accepted as dogma. In a more general manner, the Church placed itself in an entirely contradictory situation on the theological plane. The reduction of the sexual act to the status of a highly circumscribed juridical concept, the systematic exclusion of all forms of heterodox conjugal love, and the extension of the purely carnal dimension of conjugal relations, all testified to an unprecedented misreading of the spiritual vocation of marriage, which was reiterated so incessantly and with such futility by Catholic theology.

But these were not the only effects of the canonical reaction of the twentieth century.

By placing itself on the bandwagon of psychoanalysis, the Church relocated impotence within the psychological landscape, where the most diverse forms of sexual disorder and aberration bloom side by side. To the list of reasons for non-consummation, the theologians now added 'psychopathic continence, neurosis caused by onanism, sexual neuropathy . . .'

These unindividuated neuroses did not however bear any

taint of ignominy. But what about those deviations which, carefully defined by psychoanalysis, broached the areas of sexual psychopathy? 'Hyperaesthesia, sexual fetishism, sadism, homosexuality, autosexualism (narcissism) and other unnatural sexual tendencies' became so many clues which had the status of evidence. And in addition to these vices and defects which contributed irresistibly to the suspicion of impotence, there was, according to Œsterle, that of 'a sexual life rendered abnormal either through excess or insufficiency':

The arguments from assumption can be very strong, for example in the case of homosexuality. Thus in one case a dispensation was granted on the grounds of non-consummation, despite the assertions of the homosexual wife that consummation had occurred hundreds of times. Which is why in this type of trial it is very important to discover the hidden motives for non-consummation.

This bizarre conjunction of ecclesiastical authority and psychoanalysis reinforced the inquisitorial power of the Church judges in a spectacular manner. The investigation into the private life of the couple could now claim to be based on scientific principles.

Onto these reactionary theoretical foundations was grafted an improper and secretive procedural method – that of collecting evidence in the absence of the parties concerned. Contrary to the practice in other kinds of matrimonial lawsuit, the judge was no longer required to place the results of the enquiry at the disposal of the parties concerned (canon 1858–1859). Moreover, the cross-examination of the partners was punctuated by an obsessively precise litany of inquisitive questions, and witnesses were examined within the classical framework of the *septima manus*: 'What signs of affection did the couple display towards each other before the marriage, on their wedding day, and thereafter? Did they share the same bedroom and consummate the marriage? Do you know why the marriage has not been consummated?'

The investigations carried out in the course of the trial fitted clearly into the framework of modern canonical reaction. For all that these procedures were inquisitorial and secret, they nevertheless enjoyed a resounding publicity. Obviously, this was no longer the explosive and noisy publicity which formerly surged through the masses during an impotence trial. The sociological context no longer lent itself to such theatricality. But, as if by way of compensation, the Church now took to organising another kind of publicity, more discreet but more effective and organised, which was aimed at the familial and socio-professional milieu of the accused. Until the eighteenth century, legal proceedings for impotence directly involved only the litigants themselves. In modern times, relatives, friends and neighbours are all actively implicated and solicited.

At the end of these ordeals, the medical examination still lay in wait for the couple. This has remained the determining feature of the investigation. Of course, civil imprisonment is no longer imposed upon partners who refuse to submit to examination. In the event of refusal, however, the defaulter 'will be warned as to the legal consequences of his refusal'. As in civil law, moral pressure is used to replace physical force.

As far as the physical examination of the woman is concerned, the modern canonical reaction destroyed the two arguments which had formerly been able to resist it: the concern about indecency was regarded as no more than a redundant scruple, and uncertainties as to the existence of the hymen were regarded as pointless sophistry. Canon 1976 stated categorically that the proof afforded by the female examination was still required. However, a certain element of doubt persisted, and the hymen was again to become the subject of a discreet but nonetheless genuine controversy – on 2 August 1921 the Holy Rota admitted openly that 'virginity is a state so difficult to prove that even the proof by physical examination may be considered to be of minor significance.'

Such examinations nevertheless continued to take place, and many reports bear witness to the confusion of the experts.

As for male medical examinations, the contents of reports no longer rested on a straightforward assessment of the physical attributes of the accused, but now contained a formidable amount of speculative detail about the origins of the impotence in question. In the search for explanations, it often proved necessary to infer an 'abnormal' sex life, sexual excesses in youth or a propensity for sodomy. 'Unnatural copulation in the buccal aperture (mouth) or the inappropriate orifice (anus) of the wife' provided a means of accounting for non-consummation (*copula contra nature in ore aut in vase indebito*). Finally, the methods resorted to in the course of these examinations were often rather extreme. At least this is what we may surmise from a somewhat peculiar directive issued by the Holy Office, which decreed on 2 August 1929 that 'to obtain sperm, it is not permitted to resort directly to masturbation'!

Thus do four centuries of history bring us full circle, back to our original point of departure. Doubtless the institution of divorce and the relatively recent legalisation of separation on the grounds of mutual consent have partly resolved the problem and established important safety valves. The real problem however is that impotence trials still exist today. For although time may effect certain modifications, it erases nothing. The structures of thought and the myths remain as a powerful force of inertia. As a product of the myth of virility, the impotence trial does not seem to be a species in danger of extinction.

The problem which this book raises is insoluble without recourse to the unilateral breaking of the conjugal bond. To agree to debate impotence in the first place is to trigger off a poisonous chain of logic; it is to condemn oneself to a determinism whose end result was the institution of trial by congress. But the refusal to engage upon such a path should not be made in a nineteenth-century spirit. It should not proceed from any puritanism or concern for legal efficiency. Rather it should be formulated in the absolute, in categorical terms. Any sane appreciation of the problem must rest upon a straightforward rejection of the impotence trial, a visceral rejection, obeying the same imperative which urges us to drive back racism in any of its forms. For, in a vicious circle, the impotence trial is determined according to criteria which in turn engender intolerance and discrimination against individuals who, supposedly lacking in virility, have nevertheless created a certain kind of 'living space', and evolved a certain arrangement with the world. Is it any coincidence that, from Sparta to Nuremberg, the most disastrous ideologies have been those founded largely upon a coherent mythology of virility? The analogy is neither forced nor gratuitous: to condemn an individual in the name of sexual normalisation is to issue an untenable dictate, any refutation of which necessarily expresses itself through a language and a dialectic which derive from the Enlightenment. Must we continue to condemn to silence those who, by virtue of an ill-matched marriage, are exposed to sexual misery? If so, the trap is laid, and the fatal mechanism activated.

Bibliography

Note on sources. In this translated edition, detailed references have been deleted from the text. Exact sources for quoted material, as well as details of manuscripts, factums and memoirs in the *Bibliothèque Nationale* and the *Archives Nationales* in Paris, can be found in the original French edition: *Le Tribunal de l'Impuissance* (Editions du Seuil, Paris, 1979). This bibliography is a list of the major sources quoted in the text.

Anne Robert (pseudonym of Louis Servin), *Quatre Livres des arrests et choses jugées par la cour*, Paris, 1627.

Arrerac, Jean d', *La Philosophie civile et d'estat, divisée en l'Irénarchie et la Polémarchie*, Bordeaux, 1598.

Bayle, Pierre, 'Quellenec', 'Parthenay', 'Portugal', in *Dictionnaire historique et critique*, Paris, 1715.

Bignon, Jérôme, *Liber legis salicae*, Paris, 1665.

Bodin, Jean, *La République ou l'Art de gouverner un Estat*, Lyons, 1693 (1st edition, Paris, 1575).

Boileau, Jacques, *De l'abus des nuditez de gorge*, Paris, 1675.

Boniface, Hyacinthe de, *Arrests notables de la cour de parlement de Provence*, Paris, 1670.

Boucher d'Argis, Antoine Gaspard, *Principes sur la nullité du mariage pour cause d'impuissance, par M . . ., avocat au Parlement, avec le traité du président Bouhier sur les procédures . . .*, Paris, 1756.

Bouhier, Jean, *Traité des moyens qui sont en usage en France pour la preuve de l'impuissance de l'homme et quelques pièces curieuses sur le même sujet*, Paris, 1756.

Boursault, Edme, *Lettres nouvelles*.

Brantôme (Pierre de Bourdeille, seigneur de), *Vie des dames galantes*, Paris, 1947.

Briand, Joseph et Chaude, J.-S., *Manuel de médecine légale*, 7th edition, Paris, 1863 (1st edition, Paris, 1821).

Brillon, Pierre Jacques, *Dictionnaire des arrests ou jurisprudence universelle des parlements et autres tribunaux de France*, Paris, 1711.

Brunet, Gustave, *Le Nouveau Siècle de Louis XIV ou choix de chansons historiques et satiriques, de 1634 à 1712*, Paris, 1857.

Choppin, René, *Œuvres*, Vol. 4, *Traité de la police ecclésiastique*, Paris, 1662–1667.

De Barry, père Paul, *La Mort de Paulin et d'Alexis, illustres amants de la mère de Dieu, et leurs lettres à diverses personnes sur des sujets bien importants . . .*, Lyons, 1658.

Demey, Julien, *La Notion actuelle du devoir conjugal et le But du mariage devant les tribunaux civils et les officialités*, Paris, 1931.

Desmaisons, François Guillaume, *Nouveau Recueil d'arrests et réglemens du parlement de Paris*, Paris, 1733 (1st edition, 1697).

Diderot and D'Alembert, 'Impuissance', in *Encyclopédie*, Paris, 1777.

Du Laurens, André, *Les Œuvres de M. André Du Laurens, sieur de Ferrières, revues et traduites en françois par M. Théophile Gelée, médecin ordinaire de la ville de Dieppe*, Rouen, 1639 (1st edition, Paris, 1621).

Duval, Jacques, *Traité des hermaphrodits, parties génitales, accouchemens des femmes . . .*, Paris, 1880 (1st edition, Rouen, 1612).

Fevret, Charles, *Traité de l'abus et du vray sujet des appellations qualifiées de ce nom d'abus*, Dijon, 1654.

Flandrin, J. L., *Les Amours paysannes (XVIe-XIXe siècle)*, Paris, 1975.

Fodéré, François Emmanuel, 'Impuissance', in *Traité de médecine légale et d'hygiène publique ou de police de santé, adapté aux codes de l'Empire français et aux connaissances actuelles*, Vol. 1, Paris, 1813.

Garnier, Charles Georges, *Code du divorce, contenant l'explication familière des moyens et de la manière d'exécuter la loi du divorce, dans tous les cas où le divorce est permis*, Paris, 1792.

Gayot de Pitival, François, *Causes célèbres et intéressantes avec les jugements qui y sont décidés*, Paris, 1743.

Gerbais, Jean, *Traité du pouvoir de l'Église et des princes sur les empeschemens de mariage*, Paris, 1646.

Guillemeau, Jacques, *Œuvres de chirurgie*, edition of 1649.

Henri de Suze, cardinal d'Ostie, Hostiensis, *Summa aurea ad vetustissimos codices summa fide diligentiaque nunc primum collata adque ad innumeris erriribus, quibus scatebat hactenus, repurgata.*

Héricourt, Louis de, *Les Loix ecclésiastiques de France dans leur ordre naturel et une analyse des livres de droit canonique conférez avec les usages de l'Église gallicane*, Paris, 1714.

Hostiensis, voir Henri de Suze.

Hotman, Antoine, *Traité de la dissolution du mariage par l'impuissance et froideur de l'homme ou de la femme*, Paris, 1581.

Joubert, *Erreurs populaires touchant la médecine et le régime de santé*, Rouen, 1600–1601 (1st edition, Bordeaux, 1579).

Juvernay, Pierre, *Discours particulier contre les femmes débraillées de ce temps*, par Pierre Juvernay, prestre parisien, Paris, 1637.

Lamoignon, Chrétien François de, *Plaidoyé sur le congrès*, Paris, 1680.

Le Ridant, Pierre, *Traité sur le mariage*, 1754.

– *Code matrimonial ou Recueil des édits, ordonnances et déclarations sur le mariage, avec les décisions les plus importantes sur cette matière*, Paris, 1766.

– *Code matrimonial*, Paris, 1770.

Le Semelier, père Jean Laurent, *Conférences ecclésiastiques de Paris sur le mariage*, Paris, 1713.

Linguet, Simon Nicolas Henri, 'Légitimité du divorce justifiée par les Saintes Écritures, par les Pères, par les conciles . . .', Brussels, 1789.

Marais, Mathieu, *Journal et Mémoires sur la Régence et le règne de Louis XV (1715–1737)*, Paris, 1864.

Papon, Jean, *Recueil d'arrests notables des cours souveraines de France*, Paris, 1565.

– *Instrument du premier notaire de Jean Papon, conseiller du roy et lieutenant du baillage de forest*, Lyons, 1626.

Paré, Ambroise, *Toutes les œuvres*, Paris, 1585.

Peleus, Julien, *Les Plaidoyers de maistre Julien Peleus, advocat en parlement et au conseil de sa majesté*, Paris, 1614.

Polman, chanoine Jean, *Le Chancre ou Couvre-Sein féminin, ensemble, le voile ou couvre-chef féminin*, Douay, 1635.

Pothier, Robert Joseph, *Traité du contrat de mariage*, Paris, 1768.

Puymisson, Jacques, *Plaidoyez*, Rouen, 1627.

Roulliard, Sébastien, *Les Reliefs forenses*, Paris, 1610.

– *Capitulaire ou Recueil des principaux chefs du procès d'entre le seigneur baron d'Argenton . . . appelant . . . et Dame Magdeleine de La Chastre, sa femme, poursuivant la dissolution de leur mariage, intimée.*

Roussel, Michel, *Historia pontificiae juridictionis*, Paris, 1636.

Sainte-Beuve, Jacques de, *Résolution de plusieurs cas de conscience touchant la morale et la discipline de l'Église*, Paris, 1689.

Sanchez, père Tomàs, *Aphorismi Thomae Sanchez de matrimonio*, Andomari, 1629.

Sauval, Henri, *La Chronique scandaleuse de Paris, chronique des mauvais lieux* (from a manuscript of 1722), Paris, 1909.

Saviard, Barthélemy, *Nouveau Recueil d'observations chirurgicales*, Paris, 1702.

Soefve, Lucien, *Nouveau Recueil de plusieurs questions notables tant de droit que de coutume, jugées par arrests d'audiences du parlement de Paris, depuis 1640 jusqu'à présent*, Paris, 1682.

Tagereau, Vincent, *Discours sur l'impuissance de l'homme et de la femme auquel est déclaré ce que c'est qu'impuissance empeschant et séparant le mariage, comment elle se cognoist et ce qui doit estre observé aux procès de séparation pour cause d'impuissance, conformément aux saincts canons et décrets et à ce qu'en ont escrit les théologiens et canonistes*, Paris, 1611.

Tallemant des Réaux, *Historiettes pour servir à l'histoire du XVIIe siècle*, edition of 1861.

Thiers, abbé Jean Baptiste, *Traité des superstitions*, Paris, 1679.

Venette, Nicolas, *La Génération de l'homme ou Tableau de l'amour conjugal considéré dans l'état de mariage*, Parma, 1696 (1st edition 1685).

Voltaire, 'Impuissance', in *Dictionnaire philosophique*, Paris, 1879.

Zacchia, Paolo, *Pauli Zacchiae romani totius status ecclesiastici proto-medici generalis, quaestionum medico-legalium*, Lugduni, 1726.

La Courtisane déchiffrée, dédiée aux dames vertueuses de ce temps, Paris, 1617.